Sports Nutrition for Endurance Athletes

CONTENTS

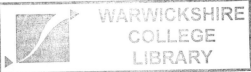

CONTENTS

This book is dedicated to all endurance athletes, and to the enhancement of their health, athletic accomplishments, and enjoyment of their sport.

I would like to thank publisher Rick Rundall and editor Amy Sorrells of VeloPress for their interest in publishing a nutrition book for endurance athletes, and for asking me to write this book. Thank you to Amy Sorrells for her input in the development of the book. Thanks to Jill Redding for her editorial expertise, and thank you to managing editor Renee Jardine for all her support and work on the final completion of this book.

Thank you also to all the athletes and clients who have shared their own athletic experiences with me over the past eighteen years, and who have allowed me to share my sports nutrition knowledge with them. And thank you to all my colleagues and friends who offered their support and encouragement during the writing and completion of this book.

INTRODUCTION

A Guide to Using This Book

Food is one of life's greatest pleasures, and chances are that you are reading this book because your training program and competition goals provide you with a worthy challenge, enjoyment, and great satisfaction. Accomplished endurance athletes appreciate that the daily food choices they make are highly interconnected with how they train and recover. Ultimately, consuming a quality training diet allows you to make the most of each training session and subsequently positively impacts your performance during competition.

Sports Nutrition for Endurance Athletes is designed for the endurance athlete interested in the everyday application of respected, cutting-edge sports nutrition science. Whether you are a seasoned marathon runner, competitive cyclist, or interested in completing your first triathlon, providing your hard-working body with the proper food choices, consumed in the right amounts at the right times, forms a solid foundation for your training and competition goals.

The quality training diet outlined and described in this book is designed to optimize your recovery on a daily basis so that you can continue to train at your highest level and progress within your sport. Eating the proper foods and fluids while training and competing provides the fuel you need to sustain you through an endurance training bike ride or run, endurance cross-country ski events, long swim sessions, an Ironman triathlon, and an adventure race. Choosing the most optimal foods for your sport can keep your body at a healthy weight and your immune system strong. Sound nutrition habits will also sustain you throughout the stages of your athletic career and goals, and help maintain good health throughout your life.

Sports Nutrition for Endurance Athletes has several unique features. First, it is designed to be a practical book, and provides a bridge between sports nutrition science and real life application of practical nutrition guidelines. In addition to the chapters that outline nutrition guidelines for good health and the latest in sports nutrition, specific nutrition advice for several popular endurance sports is included. To assist you in improving your sports nutrition knowledge and taking practical steps to adopting these nutrition guidelines, this book has been divided into three parts.

Part I, The Daily Training Diet, emphasizes that good training and performance begins with a solid nutrition foundation of quality food choices. A quality diet consisting of the highest nutrient choices on a daily basis supports good health in both training and competition. Guidelines for optimal hydration and a well-balanced intake of vitamins and minerals and other important nutrients are provided.

Part II, Training Nutrition, provides very specific nutrition guidelines outlining how to eat after training for the most optimal recovery so that you can complete your desired training sessions on a daily basis. What you consume before and during training can assist you in meeting your fuel and fluid needs as closely as possible. Because a lean, strong body is so important to endurance sports, body composition concerns regarding weight management, body fat loss, and muscle building are provided. A full chapter on meal planning is included to assist you in putting together the sports diet that fits your training goals and lifestyle. Because endurance athletes have a great interest in supplements, a full chapter reviewing the current scientific data on ergogenic aids is also provided.

Part III, Sport Specific Nutrition Plans, outlines nutrition plans for the following sports: triathlon, road cycling and mountain biking, distance running, swimming, cross-country skiing, and adventure racing. These chapters will address the unique nutritional strategies for training and competing in each sport. Each chapter also highlights an aspect of sports nutrition that is relevant to that particular sport, such as nutrition guidelines for training at altitude and exercising in extremely hot and cold environments.

I trust and hope that the information provided in this book will enhance your athletic accomplishments and enjoyment of your sport.

—*Monique Ryan, MS, RD*

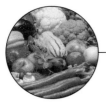

THE DAILY TRAINING DIET

Building a Healthy Sports Nutrition Foundation

*F*or endurance athletes, consuming the optimal balance of foods required is primarily about achieving their best athletic performance. But with all the attention that nutrition receives in the popular press and from health care professionals, it is also clear that what you eat can have a significant impact on your health. Part I provides you with nutrition guidelines upon which to build your training diet and to promote optimal health and a strong immune system. You will learn about the most nutritious sources of carbohydrates, protein, and fat to consume for training and health, and be provided with the guidelines necessary for meeting the fluid, vitamin, and mineral intakes required to build the foundation of a cutting-edge sports diet and good health.

chapter 1

FLUID FIRST

Daily Hydration Essentials

F luid is the most essential nutrient for endurance athletes. When watching top athletes perform, you may have been struck by their obvious sweat losses. Adequate hydration is crucial for both general well being and athletic performance. In fact, even though it deserves top priority from any athlete, daily water intake is often a secondary nutrition consideration and many athletes frequently fall short on consumption of the most important nutrient in our daily diet. Endurance athletes should not only pay attention to their fluid intake while cycling, running, skiing, and swimming, but also throughout the day.

Much marketing fuss has been made about the optimal fluids that athletes require. But before the plethora of sports related drinks arrived and flooded the market, there was simply water. Water is basic and unpretentious and flows naturally into your active life with no packaging or gimmicks attached. Don't take water for granted, as it is an essential part of your daily training diet. Just as you don't want to arrive to training and competition with a low fuel tank, your fluid stores should be topped off as well.

Water is both a significant part of your body and plays an integral role in its optimal functioning, whether you are training or not. Anywhere from 60 to 70 percent of your body weight is water. Muscle tissue is also high in fluid content, with about 70 to 75 percent of your muscle comprised of water. Water is stored in many body compartments, and it moves freely between these various spaces. Much of your body's water is stored inside your body cells, giving them their shape and form. Water also provides structure to body parts, consequently protecting important tissues, such as your brain and spinal cord, and lubricating your joints.

Endurance athletes will appreciate that fluid is also the main component of their blood. Blood carries oxygen, hormones, and nutrients such as glucose to your cells and is linked to important body fuel and nutrient stores such as protein, carbohydrates, and electrolytes. The protein content of blood, muscle, and other tissues also binds water in those tissues. Muscle glycogen holds a considerable amount of water, and water removes lactic acid from exercising muscles, which can be an advantage to endurance athletes. Water is involved in digestion through saliva and stomach secretions, and it eliminates waste products through urine and sweat. Water is essential for all your senses, such as hearing, sight, and sound, to function properly.

Clearly the role water plays in maintaining your overall health is extremely important. That's why you can't live without water for more than a few days. But the role that water plays in your performance is also essential. As the primary component of sweat, water plays a major role in body temperature regulation. You are able to maintain a constant body temperature under various environmental conditions by continually making adjustments to either gain or lose heat. Your fluid balance is the result of your intake versus output. Intake is the net result of the water and hydrating fluids we consume, water in some of the foods we eat, and the metabolic water produced by the body. At rest, urine output represents our greatest losses, while sweating during exercise can incur significant fluid losses, especially for the endurance athlete. Fluid is also lost in feces and the air you exhale. Warm or humid weather, living in a dry climate, or living at altitude all increase fluid losses. Traveling, especially by plane, can boost water loss. In general your body loses about 64–80 ounces (8–10 cups) of fluid daily through the urine, feces, skin, and lungs. Your daily water requirements are based upon the amount of calories you consume. Your body requires one millileter of water per calorie. Endurance athletes who consume 4,000 calories daily require 4,000 millileters of fluid, or approximately 16 cups of fluid daily.

WHAT ABOUT SWEAT?

When you train, heat is a major byproduct of your working muscles. As this heat builds up, your body temperature rises. Water then acts as a coolant to keep the body from overheating. During exercise, sweating is the body's primary mechanism for getting rid of excess heat. Sweat losses can easily reach anywhere from 16 to 32 ounces, and sometimes even 48 ounces per hour depending on environmental conditions and the individual athlete.

One of water's functions in the body is to maintain adequate blood supply to the skin. This blood transfers heat to the environment through sweating. When sweat evaporates it cools the skin, blood, and your body's inner core. Athletes who are in top shape actually sweat more than their sedentary counterparts, rendering their fluid needs quite high. So while it may appear that your tolerance to training in the heat improves, your fluid requirements go up.

Though sweating does the important job of keeping your body cool, the resulting minor to large fluid losses can impair your athletic performance during both training and competition. Even losing as little as 2 percent of your body weight through sweat can impair your ability to exercise. With sweating, blood volume is decreased and greater demands are placed upon your cardiovascular system, which reduces your ability to take in and utilize oxygen. Muscular endurance ability is also impaired with dehydration and your heart rate may increase at a given level of intensity. When fluid losses through sweat are not replaced, your body temperature rises further and exercise becomes harder. Clearly, not meeting your fluid needs hinders your athletic goals.

Unfortunately thirst is not a very good indicator of the amount of fluid that your body requires, during exercise or at rest. Some early signs and symptoms of

1.1

PHYSIOLOGICAL EFFECTS AND SYMPTOMS OF DEHYDRATION

PHYSIOLOGICAL EFFECTS OF DEHYDRATION	SYMPTOMS OF DEHYDRATION
Decreased:	**Mild dehydration:**
Blood volume	Dark urine
Cardiac output	Decreased appetite
Skin blood flow	Fatigue
Sweat rate	Heat intolerance
Urine output	Light-headedness
	Small amount of urine
Increased:	Thirst
Body temperature	
Heart rate	**Severe dehydration:**
	Delirium
	Difficulty swallowing
	Dry, shriveled skin
	Muscle spasms
	Sunken eyes

dehydration are light-headedness, headaches, decreased appetite, darkly colored urine, and fatigue. When you are thirsty, you have already lost 1 percent of your body weight through fluid loss. When fluid losses reach about 2 to 4 percent of your body weight, increased thirst and symptoms such as irritability and nausea may occur. At losses of 5 to 6 percent of body weight there will be an increase in heart rate and breathing regulation, and body temperature regulation will be significantly impaired. Table 1.1 describes some the physiological effects and symptoms of dehydration. Pay attention to how you feel during the day. An annoying headache may indicate the need to up your fluid intake.

DAILY HYDRATION ESSENTIALS

It is essential that you stay on top of your fluid needs by drinking a minimum of 60–80 ounces (8–10 cups) of fluid daily. Try to drink on a schedule of 8 ounces every hour. Water should comprise about half of your daily fluid intake, but you can also receive hydration benefits from non-caffeinated fluids. Hydrating choices include juice, dairy milk, soy milk, and various sports nutrition supplements. Endurance athletes with very high energy requirements can consume high calorie drinks such as juices and smoothies to assist them in meeting their fluid, carbohydrate, and energy needs. Caffeinated beverages can be incorporated into your diet in reasonable amounts, but should not be your first choice for hydration purposes. Overdoing the caffeine may interfere with your sleep patterns and make you nervous and jittery. Excess caffeine may also act as a mild diuretic shortly after you drink a caffeine-containing beverage. However, overall, new research suggests that caffeine-containing beverages are not as dehydrating as they were once thought to be, and can be included in moderate amounts with other fluids in the diet.

Table 1.2 reviews daily hydration strategies. Improving your fluid intake on a daily basis merely takes practice. One top cyclist made a point of taking a full water bottle with her everywhere she went. She liked purchasing one- or two-quart bottles of water and refilling them throughout the day to keep track of her fluid intake.

Just as a heart rate monitor gives you feedback on your exercise intensity, you can monitor your hydration status by checking the color and quantity of your urine. Clear urine reflects adequate fluid intake, while darker urine indicates that you need to step

---

1.2

DAILY HYDRATION STRATEGIES

- Start your day with hydration in mind. Consume liquids such as juice, dairy, or soy milk at breakfast. Drink 8–16 ounces of water or hydrating fluid when you start your day, especially when you consume caffeinated beverages in the morning.

- Keep caffeine-containing beverages to moderate amounts.

- Carry water with you at all times: when you drive or commute, at work or school, and wherever the opportunity to drink presents itself.

- Fit juices, milk, or soy milk into all your meals or snacks.

- Spruce up your water with lemon, lime, or a small amount of juice for flavor.

- Consume any serving of alcohol with a full 8–12 ounces of hydrating fluid.

- Consider consuming foods high in fluid such as fruits and vegetables, cooked cereals, and yogurt.

- Consume 24 ounces of fluid two hours before exercise and 8–16 ounces of fluid 30 minutes before exercise to ensure adequate hydration prior to exercise.

up your fluid intake. Urine tends to be more concentrated when you first wake up, but should be clearer throughout the day. You should urinate at least four full bladders every day. Certain vitamin supplements can darken urine, so volume rather than color may be a better indicator of hydration status if you take these products.

Besides meeting your daily hydration requirements, consuming a planned amount of fluids before, during, and after exercise can have a positive effect on your training and competition efforts. Sports drinks are also a very important fluid consideration for endurance athletes. These topics will be covered in Chapter 5, Eating for Training and Competition.

Focusing and practicing to improve your daily fluid intake is definitely worthwhile. Athletes who have developed techniques for increasing their fluid intake have consistently found that improved hydration resulted in enhanced recovery and higher energy levels. Improving your hydration levels is really very simple. Just plan ahead and make sure that water and other hydrating fluids are available for consumption throughout the day. This will ensure that you begin your training sessions with a well-hydrated body.

ELECTROLYTES

Sodium is one of the major electrolytes in the body and the one of greatest interest to the endurance athlete. Sodium is found outside the body's cells and helps to regulate blood pressure and blood volume. The concentration of sodium in your body plays a role in regulating the distribution of fluids and nutrients between the inside and outside of the cells. Your body has a fairly complicated system of regulating your sodium and fluid balance between your fluid intake and fluid losses, and the balance of other electrolytes including potassium and chloride. Sodium is also critical for nerve impulse transmission and muscle contraction, and is essential in maintaining a normal blood pressure.

Most importantly for endurance athletes, sodium is lost in sweat. The body can conserve how much sodium is lost in sweat when sweat rates are high. Any sodium losses can then be replaced through your daily diet. However, there are some strategies designed to optimize sodium levels during ultraendurance exercise that you may have to consider, especially when training and racing in hot and humid conditions. These recommendations will be covered in Chapter 5. Sodium can also play an important role in your recovery from exercise, which will be covered in Chapter 4, Eating for Optimal Recovery.

While you may have unique sodium requirements for training and racing, your daily sodium requirements are more than adequately met by the typical North American diet. Sodium is found in small amounts in most natural foods, but the processing so prevalent in our diet has added significant amounts of sodium to our daily intake. Because of health concerns, many individuals limit their sodium intake. Excess sodium may exacerbate high blood pressure and interfere with calcium balance.

Adults require a minimum of 500 milligrams of sodium in their daily diet and the upper recommended intake is 2,400 milligrams per day. But it is not unusual for individuals to obtain several thousand milligrams of sodium in their everyday diet, mainly through consumption of processed foods and table salt or sodium chloride of which 40 percent is sodium. Be reasonable with your sodium and salt intake to minimize any health risks. However, as will be covered in later chapters, there may be specific athletic situations in which increasing sodium intake may benefit your athletic performance.

ALCOHOL

It is very possible that alcohol is a moderate part of your current lifestyle. But as an athlete you should use alcohol sensibly, as this drink does not play any important role in your recovery and could have detrimental effects upon your performance. Obviously alcohol abuse can affect your health and that of others by contributing to liver cirrhosis and drunk driving. But let's take a look at the implications of alcohol in regards to your training diet and athletic performance.

Filtered, Bottled, or Tap?

While the tap water in the United States is very safe, many American consumers have purchased home filtration systems and consumed more than 5 billion gallons of bottled water in the year 2000 alone. Currently, the Environmental Protection Agency (EPA) estimates that 90 percent of the country's drinking water is safe.

Tap water does contain substances other than water. Depending on where you live it can provide varying levels of minerals such as calcium, sodium, magnesium, iron, zinc, lead, and mercury. While calcium may be a beneficial mineral obtained from water, lead is not. As a health-minded athlete and consumer, you may also be concerned about microbial contamination and pesticide residues in water.

Tap water is regulated under the strict standards of the EPA. Your local water municipality is required to supply you with an annual report and tests for microbes several times daily. You can also contact your local water municipality to obtain the names and numbers of certified testing labs to have the water from your own tap checked. Levels of lead and copper in your water may be higher than official reports due to leaching from household plumbing and faucets. If you prefer, filtered water may be a viable option. You may also determine that bottled water is a convenient option for reaching your recommended daily water intake.

Both water filter systems and bottled water can be certified by an independent organization called the National Sanitation Foundation (NSF). The NSF sets standards for and certifies water filtration systems. Their website at www.nsf.org lists filters and the contaminants that the filter is certified to reduce in your water. Be sure to follow the manufacturer's directions for replacement of the filter cartridge.

Bottled water is currently regulated by the Food and Drug Administration (FDA), but receives less scrutiny than tap water, which is regulated under stricter standards by the EPA. Water testing is required once weekly for microbes. Testing for contaminants and chemicals is also done more frequently on tap water than bottled water. That's why it is also a good idea to look for brands of bottled water that maintain the NSF certification. In order to maintain this certification, water bottlers must send daily samples for microbial testing to an independent lab and maintain records of filter changes and other quality checks. You can also determine if your brand of water is NSF certified by visiting the website mentioned above. ■

While alcohol is a drug, it provides calories just as foods do and makes for fairly caloric beverages. As far as your body is concerned, alcohol is merely a bunch of empty calories. Beer and wine contain only small amounts of carbohydrates and only trace amounts of protein, vitamins, and minerals. One-half ounce of pure ethanol is the equivalent of one drink that equals 12 ounces of beer (150 calories), 4 ounces of wine (100 calories), and 1.25 ounces of liquor (100 calories).

Despite originating from fermented carbohydrates, alcohol is metabolized in your body as fat. Alcohol byproducts are converted into fatty acids, which are stored in your liver and sent to your bloodstream. Much has been made of alcohol's protective effects against heart disease. But while moderate amounts may raise the desirable and protective high-density lipoprotein (HDL) cholesterol, too much alcohol may actually increase your risk of heart disease. Depositing extra fat in your abdominal area, which alcohol is prone to do, increases a measurement referred to as a waist-to-hip ratio. This high level of abdominal fat is often associated with increased levels of the harmful blood fats called triglycerides, which, when combined with a low amount of the good cholesterol (HDL), makes for a health profile associated with an increased risk of heart disease. Consumed in excess over a long period, alcohol may elevate blood pressure, increase the risk of stroke and certain cancers, and of course result in liver damage.

Too much alcohol too soon after training and racing can impede recovery. Though you may rehydrate well after training, alcohol is a diuretic that causes your body to lose more fluid than it takes in. That's why you need to replace losses even after drinking moderate amounts of alcohol. Alcohol may also interfere with glycogen synthesis. Athletes with soft tissue damage or bruising may also want to consider that alcohol is a blood vessel dilator. Consuming alcohol after exercise may aggravate swelling or bleeding and impair healing. These types of injuries are usually treated with ice, which is designed to constrict blood flow to the injured parts.

Excessive alcohol consumed the night before, or alcohol consumed shortly before training, can impair fine motor ability and coordination, increase risk of dehydration, and impair fuel stores. Reaction times are delayed, as your brain's ability to process information is impaired. Know your limits and how they change with your training and fitness level. How fast you metabolize alcohol varies with body size. Average-sized men metabolize slightly less than one drink per hour, while smaller men and women take longer to metabolize this amount.

Consuming alcohol during cold weather is not advisable. While alcohol does increase your sense of warmth by increasing blood flow to your skin, this effect could actually result in considerable heat loss. Safer and more warming beverages would be hot cider, hot cocoa, and hot tea with honey.

Alcohol can be a small part of a healthy sports diet, but drink in sensible amounts. Have a large glass of water with each drink. Consider that your top priority as an athlete is recovery. Too much alcohol can compromise how effectively you recover.

chapter 2

THE DAILY TRAINING DIET

Making Food Choices for Optimal Performance and Good Health

THE IMPORTANCE OF YOUR DAILY DIET

Because you regularly participate in endurance training for your sport, your daily food intake has a significant impact on your health and recovery. Whatever level of your sport you train at and whatever level you wish to attain, the training hours you put in on a weekly basis require that you choose the right amount and types of foods at the best times to replace the fuel stores that you burn for energy. It is this daily recovery that will allow you to complete the desired training sessions and ultimately arrive for the competition in the best form possible. You must meet the nutritional demands placed upon your body by your training in order to derive the maximum benefit from your program.

Trained bodies also benefit from premium fuel to stay healthy. If you suffer from lackluster training days, injuries, and frequent infections such as colds, you may not be making the highest quality fuel choices possible. Your body uses more than forty different nutrients for optimal functioning. Take a sensible approach to planning your diet by consuming a wide variety of foods in moderate amounts for the full spectrum of nutrients they provide. When it comes to nutrition, endurance athletes should keep the big picture in mind and downplay the "good" versus "bad" food concept, and adopt the philosophy that foods should taste good as well as fuel your body. Your high energy needs for endurance training leave a reasonable amount of room for favorites.

Variety, Moderation, Balance, and Quality

Endurance athletes should appreciate that foods are complex and usually provide more than a single nutrient. While a morning glass of orange juice may be an excellent source of vitamin C, it also provides energy in the form of carbohydrates and is an excellent source of potassium as well. Lean red meat is a good source of protein, but also provides the valuable minerals of iron and zinc. Eating a variety of foods at meals and snacks allows these nutrients to work together to improve the quality of your meals and overall diet. While a variety of quality foods are available in the North American diet, excessive amounts of highly processed foods are also available. Nutrient dense foods should be emphasized in your diet as they provide a higher nutritional value than comparable processed foods in similar serving sizes. For your health and to prevent chronic disease, it is best if processed foods are not a mainstay in your diet. But when you do choose a wholesome and varied diet the majority of the time, there is still room for enjoyable foods that may not be as high in nutrients.

It takes planning and thought to put together a balanced diet high in nutrients. One way to regard and organize nutrition and your diet is through food groups. Often foods are grouped according to their carbohydrate, protein, and fat content, as the proper balance of these nutrients supports good health and gives an endurance athlete the optimal balance of fuel for training and recovery. Foods often supply one or more of these three nutrients, but can be placed into the following categories based on the predominant nutrient.

Sources of carbohydrates

Grains, breads, cereals, rice, and pasta

Fruits and fruit juices

Vegetables

Sources of protein

Milk and yogurt

Meat, poultry, fish, cheese, and eggs

Soy, dried beans, and lentils

Sources of fat

Fat, oils, nuts, and seeds

Other

Sweets and alcohol

The pie chart below provides a general guideline of how you can balance the various food groups to achieve an optimal sports diet. Of course every endurance athlete can benefit from personalized nutrition guidelines. Some individuals may prefer a heavier emphasis on fruits and vegetables in their diet than grains to obtain their daily carbohydrate intake needed for recovery. Other athletes may prefer that the majority of their protein intake be derived from more concentrated plant sources such as soy and dried beans, while some individuals may or may not prefer to have a significant amount of dairy products in their diet.

Sample Sports Diet Composition

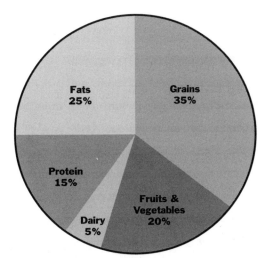

While grouping and categorizing foods can be useful for planning a healthy sports diet, it can also be an oversimplification. For example, animal protein foods provide varying levels of fat. Grains provide small amounts of protein, and milk and yogurt provide carbohydrates as well as protein.

Much speculation has been made over the optimal proportions of carbohydrates, protein, and fat for the endurance athlete. But because of the unique fuel require-ments of endurance training, it is generally recommended that your diet provide about 60 percent carbohydrates, 15 to 20 percent protein, and 20 to 25 percent fat. It is important to keep in mind that these percentages are all relative and based on consuming an adequate number of calories or energy that match your training that day. Variations in these percentages can be fine if that is what suits meeting the fuel demands of that day's training session.

First, let's take a look at some of the food choices available within these designated food groups so that you can appreciate which choices are the most nutritious. How you portion and time these foods with your training is what distinguishes your sports nutrition diet from an ordinary healthy diet. More information on timing and portioning of these fuels and how your diet replenishes your body stores will be reviewed in Chapters 4 and 5.

CARBOHYDRATES PROVIDE ENERGY

Carbohydrate foods are the foundation of an optimal diet for the endurance athlete's diet. Foods that provide carbohydrates include grains, fruits, and vegetables. Milk and yogurt are also good carbohydrate sources. Within each of these groups, some choices are more nutrient dense than others. Carbohydrates perform several important functions for the athlete. They are a quick source of energy for your daily activity. But most importantly, dietary carbohydrates replenish muscle and liver glycogen stores. Glycogen is the body's storage form of carbohydrates and is an essential fuel source for endurance training. Not adequately replenishing these glycogen stores with the proper food choices can compromise the quality of your training.

Classifying Carbohydrates: It's Not So Simple

Many athletes are familiar with the traditional classification of carbohydrates. Simple carbohydrates or sugars consist of one or two molecules, while complex carbohydrates or starches are composed of up to thousands of carbohydrate molecules joined together. What was long advised regarding these foods was that simple carbohydrates·such as fructose and sugars cause a rapid rise and subsequent fall in blood sugar that results in fatigue, and that these sugars are less nutritious. Conversely, it was maintained that complex carbohydrates resulted in a more gentle blood glucose rise and are more nutritious foods. In summary, simple carbohydrates were considered "bad" and complex carbohydrates were "good."

While this classification might seem logical, recent scientific data indicate that it is an outdated concept. What endurance athletes should truly be concerned about is the quality of the carbohydrates they consume, and they should place an emphasis on wholesome versus refined sources. Wholesome carbohydrates provide vitamins, minerals, and fiber, while refined carbohydrates are processed foods with a much lower or poor nutrient content, providing little other than carbohydrate calories. What is important to appreciate is that wholesome carbohydrates are not always complex, and refined carbohydrates are not always simple. Fruit is a simple carbohydrate packed with nutrients, while products made from complex white flour often have a much lower vitamin and mineral content. For optimal training and good health, wholesome carbohydrates are a very important component of your diet because they are higher in nutritional value.

In addition to viewing carbohydrates as wholesome or refined, they can also be categorized according to how they affect your blood sugar or blood glucose levels. The belief that simple carbohydrates cause a rapid rise in blood glucose and that complex carbohydrates cause a slower rise in blood glucose is outdated. Recent nutrition research has demonstrated that each carbohydrate food produces its own unique blood glucose profile that does not correlate with the simple versus complex classification.

The ranking system that describes the blood glucose profile of a food is referred to as the glycemic index. In this system, the blood glucose profile of 50 grams of pure glucose has been ascribed a glycemic index of 100. Other carbohydrates are tested in 50-gram doses and compared to glucose. High glycemic foods are generally considered to have a glycemic index of greater than 70. Moderate glycemic index foods are in the 50 to 70 range, and low glycemic index foods have a score of less than 50.

Table 2.1 provides a glycemic index ranking of high carbohydrate foods. Interestingly fruits generally have a low glycemic index, despite being simple carbohydrates, while potatoes, a complex carbohydrate, have a high glycemic index. Many factors influence the glycemic index of a food, including the type of fiber in the food, how the glucose molecules in the food are connected, and the form of the food.

Currently, individuals who need to control blood glucose and blood fat levels can manipulate the glycemic index to their benefit. The glycemic index can also play a role in treating a condition referred to as metabolic syndrome that is characterized by a resistance to using the body's insulin appropriately. The glycemic index has also been studied for use by endurance athletes in regards to eating before, during, and after training. These sports nutrition applications of glycemic index will be reviewed in later chapters.

2.1

GLYCEMIC INDEX OF FOODS

High Glycemic Foods	(GI > 70)
Rice, Instant	90
Potato, baked	85
Corn Flakes	83
Rice Krispies	82
Bread, wheat	78
Total cereal	76
Waffle	76
Cheerios	74
Watermelon	72
Bagel, white	72
Millet	71
Bread, white	71

Moderate Glycemic Foods	(GI 50–70)
Shredded wheat	69
Pineapple	66
Oat kernel bread	65
Couscous	65
Raisins	64
Muffin	62
Muesli	56
Oat Bran	55
Rice, brown	55
Spaghetti, durum	55
Sweet potato	54

Low Glycemic Foods	(GI < 50)
Porridge oatmeal	49
Grapefruit juice	48
Mixed grain bread	48
Peach	47
All-bran	42
Apple	38
Pear	37
Spaghetti, wholemeal	37
Kidney beans	34
Rye	34
Yogurt, fruited	33
Milk, skim	32
Lentils	29
Barley	25

Note: Values are based on a glucose rating of 100.
Source: THE GI FACTOR, Dr. Jennie Brand-Miller

Go for the Grains

Wholesome grains are good sources of carbohydrates, fiber, and B vitamins. Because they are so concentrated in carbohydrates, they are excellent choices for replenishing your body's carbohydrate stores, namely muscle and liver glycogen, which become depleted from intense and longer training sessions. Grains are easily obtained in the American diet, but unfortunately many of these choices are refined grains rather than whole grains.

For your health and your sports diet, choose whole grains whenever possible. Whole grains literally come from the entire grain that includes the endosperm, germ, and bran portion of the grain, and retain all the desirable nutrients found in whole grains. For refined grains, the bran and germ are separated from the starchy endosperm. The endosperm is then ground into flour.

Whole grains are packed with vitamins and minerals and phytochemicals, which have powerful antioxidant and disease fighting properties that you won't obtain from white bread, processed cereals, white rice, and even many "enriched" multigrain breads. Some of the phytochemicals found in whole grains include oligosaccharides, flavonoids, lignans, phytates, and saponins, many of which have powerful antioxidant properties. Whole grains also provide vitamin E and selenium. Studies have shown that regular consumption of whole grains is linked to prevention of heart disease, diabetes, and certain cancers. Surveys indicate that most Americans consume less than one serving of whole grains daily.

There are a variety of whole grains that you can include in your diet. Even just making simple changes such as having brown rice instead of white rice and whole wheat pasta rather than semolina pasta is beneficial. Buy 100-percent whole grain breads and look for "whole grain" on the health claim packages, which indicates that more than half of the weight of the product comes from whole grains. Table 2.2 provides some tips for filling your diet in with whole grains.

Athletes who are tired of the same wheat- and rice-based grain choices also have a few more adventuresome options. There are many whole grain alternatives including amaranth, kasha (buckwheat), quinoa, spelt, teff, and triticale. Table 2.3 provides a list of some top grain alternatives. They may take a bit more cooking time than pasta, rice, and potatoes, but they are nutritious and add variety to the diet. Experiment with various seasonings to further flavor these wholesome grains.

Whole grains should be an important part of your diet for the nutrients and carbohydrates they provide. But you should also place a strong emphasis on fruits and vegetables not only for their carbohydrate content, but also the great health benefits they offer. In fact, some health organizations and health researchers believe that fruits and vegetables should comprise the majority of our carbohydrate intake.

2.2

GUIDELINES FOR GETTING IN THE GRAINS

- Aim for three servings of whole grains each day. One slice or ounce of bread equals a serving and one ounce of cereal equals a serving.

- Find a whole grain cereal that you enjoy. Good choices include oatmeal or bran flakes.

- Buy breads that list 100-percent whole grain flour as the first ingredient, and for all other listed flours as well.

- Use brown rice instead of white and whole wheat pasta instead of semolina.

- Add All-bran or wheat germ with your yogurt, in smoothies, or in other cereals.

- Look for the "whole grain" health claim on the package, which indicates that more than half the weight of the product comes from whole grains.

Studies have shown that eating more fruits and vegetables can reduce your risk of heart disease, stroke, and some types of cancer. How you put together your sports diet will ultimately depend upon your food preferences, convenience, and your personal health considerations. But chances are that boosting your fruit and vegetable intake would be a healthy step in the right direction for any endurance athlete.

Plenty of Fruit

Fruits are not only excellent sources of carbohydrates but also a number of health protecting nutrients such as fiber, potassium, vitamins A and C, carotenoids, and a variety of phytochemicals. Because they are so packed with disease fighting nutrients, a high number of daily fruit servings is strongly recommended by the

WHOLE GRAIN ALTERNATIVES

Grain	Description	Tips
Amaranth	High in protein and fiber. Good source of vitamin E.	Boil and eat as a cereal. Cook 1 cup grain in 3 cups water for 1/2 hour.
Kasha (Buckwheat groats)	Excellent source magnesium and high in fiber.	Serve as a cereal, pilaf, or make pancakes. Simmer 1 part groats to 2 parts water for 15 min.
Millet	A staple in Africa. High in minerals.	Cook 1 cup grain with 2 1/4 cups water 25–30 min. Serve with meat or cook as a cereal.
Quinoa	Excellent source of B vitamins, copper, iron, and magnesium.	Can make an oatmeal-like cereal. Rinse before cooking to remove bitter coating. Cook 1 cup quinoa in 2 cups water for 20 min.
Spelt	A distant cousin to wheat. High in fiber and B vitamins.	Used to make breads and pastas. Can be used in pilafs. Cook 1 cup with 4 cups water 30–40 min.
Teff	The world's smallest grain. Rich in protein and calcium.	Serve as a hot breakfast cereal or as part of a stew. Cook 1 cup of teff in 3 cups water for 15–20 min.

American Heart Association and the American Cancer Society. Fresh fruits, dried fruits, and fruit juice can also provide the endurance athlete with a significant and concentrated source of carbohydrates.

While all fruits are nutritious, some choices are extremely nutritious. Tropical fruits such as papaya, mango, kiwifruit, and guava have wonderfully high levels of vitamin C and carotenoids, which are potent antioxidants. Carotenoids are also found in significant amounts in deep-colored fruits such as apricots, cantaloupe, and nectarines. Citrus fruits such as oranges and grapefruits are known for being great sources of vitamin C. Phytonutrients such as quercetin, ellagic acid, anthocyanins, limonin, zeaxanthin, and leutin, which appear increasingly important to maintaining good health, are also found in fruits. The best way to obtain a variety of phytonutrients is to consume a variety of fruits. Dried fruit and juices will provide the most concentrated sources of carbohydrate for athletes with higher energy needs. Dried fruit, however, will not be as great a source of vitamin C, though it may provide more minerals and fiber than fresh because it is so concentrated. Try to avoid dried fruit prepared with sulfites if you are sulfite sensitive. Sulfites are preservatives that trigger allergic reactions in some individuals. Fresh fruits are also great sources of fiber and the highest in nutrients. Table 2.4 provides a list of some top fruit choices.

Plenty of Vegetables

Like fruits, vegetables provide a wide variety of vitamins, minerals, phytonutrients, and fiber that maintain optimal health. All vegetables are good healthy choices, but some stand out nutritionally and are even more concentrated in nutrients than fruit. Color is often a good indicator of a higher nutrient content. Some stellar options include carrots, sweet potatoes, and red peppers, which are high in carotenoids. Spinach and Romaine lettuce are good leafy choices for their vitamin C, folate, and phytonutrient content. Another group of vegetables that not only contain beta-carotene and vitamin C but also the cancer fighting phytonutrients indoles, are broccoli, cauliflower, bok choy, collards, Brussels sprouts, and kale.

Each day try to consume a variety of colorful vegetables that are yellow, orange, red, and deep green. Choose large servings of vegetables when you eat at home, as it can be challenging to obtain quality vegetable choices when eating out. Buy fresh vegetables when you know you will consume them in a few days, and store them in the refrigerator crisper drawer. Frozen vegetables are a good second choice. Avoid overcooking your vegetables in order to preserve all the wonderful nutrients they contain. Table 2.4 provides a list of some top vegetable choices.

TOP FRUIT AND VEGETABLE CHOICES

Good Sources of Vitamin C	Good Sources of Carotenoids and Vitamin A
Artichoke	Apricot
Blackberries	Broccoli
Broccoli	Cantaloupe
Brussels sprouts	Carrot
Cauliflower	Guava
Grapefruit	Kale
Kiwifruit	Mango
Mango	Nectarine
Okra	Peach
Orange	Romaine lettuce
Papaya	Spinach
Peas	Sweet pepper
Pineapple	Sweet potato
Potato	Swiss chard
Strawberries	Winter squash
Tangerine	
Tomato	

THE POWER OF PROTEIN

While carbohydrates are a staple for the endurance athlete, you also need adequate amounts of protein foods to perform your best. Protein plays an important role in the growth, repair, and maintenance of muscles and other body tissues. It is also required to form hormones, enzymes, neurotransmitters, and key components of the immune system. Protein is needed for formation of hemoglobin, the substance that carries oxygen to the exercising muscles. Protein can also supply fuel for energy in the later stages of endurance exercise. Your protein intake can comprise 15 to 20 percent of your daily energy consumption. Generally athletes seem to exceed their protein intake, most likely due to large protein portions prevalent in the North American diet. But endurance athletes who restrict certain foods in attempts to limit or avoid fat intake could be at risk for consuming inadequate protein.

Protein foods are easily obtained in the North American diet. Animal protein in the form of lean meats, poultry, fish, and eggs is the most concentrated source of protein. Many of these animal proteins are also good sources of iron and zinc. High quality plant sources of protein include soy products such as tofu and tempeh, dried peas and beans, and lentils. Low fat dairy foods are also an excellent source of protein and the important mineral calcium. What is important for optimal health is

2.5

PROTEIN CONTENT OF SELECTED FOODS

Food and Portion	Protein (g)
Chicken, white, 3 oz. cooked	25
Pork, lean, 3 oz. cooked	23
Beef, lean, 3 oz. cooked	21
Tofu, firm, 4 oz.	20
White fish, 3 oz. cooked	20
Lentils, cooked, 1 cup	18
Soy milk, 1 cup	10
Milk, 8 oz.	8
Peanut butter, 2 Tbsp.	8
Cheese, 1 oz.	7

to choose lean protein sources, as this will reduce your intake of saturated fat. Table 2.5 lists the protein content of certain foods per specified portion. Try to emphasize leaner choices of red meats to limit your intake of saturated fat.

FACTS ABOUT FAT

Fat is an important part of an endurance athlete's diet. While fat is somewhat renowned for being a concentrated source of calories, it plays several key roles in keeping you healthy. Most importantly, fat is a source of nutrients known as essential fatty acids. Just as you need to obtain vitamins and minerals in your diet, you also need to obtain the essential fatty acids linoleic acid and alpha-linolenic acid from the foods you eat. Another important function of fat is its role in the transport and absorption of fat-soluble vitamins and carotenoids. Fat can also add a wonderful flavor to meals, making them more filling and satisfying.

Fat comes in several chemical forms, some healthier than others. Depending on their composition, fats are categorized as saturated or unsaturated. Unsaturated fats include both polyunsaturated and monounsaturated fats. Currently the American Heart Association sets the recommended range of fat intake at 15 to 30 percent of total calories. Exceeding this range may increase the risk of heart disease, while going below this range could result in essential fatty acid insufficiency in some individuals.

For endurance athletes, a diet in which 20 to 25 percent of the calories are supplied from fat should be appropriate. This provides adequate fat to replenish fuel stores after training, and leaves room for adequate carbohydrates and protein in the diet. However, endurance athletes with especially high calorie requirements may simply require more fat in their diet to meet their energy needs.

For prevention of heart disease, it is important to limit the amount of saturated fat you consume. Saturated fats raise the harmful low-density lipoprotein (LDL) cholesterol. This undesirable fat is found mainly in fatty animal foods such as cheese, whole milk products, fatty cuts of meat, highly processed lunch meats, butter, lard, and shortening. Palm, palm kernel, and coconut oil are three highly saturated plant oils, which can sometimes be found in processed foods and commercially baked goods.

Another group of fats that are of concern in the North American diet are trans fatty acids. Trans fatty acids are created from liquid oils that are "partially hydrogenated." Hydrogenation turns liquid corn oil into margarine sticks and increases the shelf life of commercial products that contain these altered oils. Some common sources of trans fat include cookies, crackers, and snack chips. Current data continue to verify that these fats can increase LDL cholesterol, just like saturated fat. Check labels to limit hydrogenated oils as much as possible, particularly if they are listed as one of the first several ingredients. Choose margarine that lists "liquid oil" as the first ingredient.

Unsaturated fats, both polyunsaturated and monounsaturated, can help lower LDL cholesterol when they replace saturated fat in your diet. Sources of polyunsaturated fat include corn oil, safflower oil, sunflower oil, walnuts, and sunflower seeds. These oils should comprise up to one-third of your total fat intake. Most health care professionals advocate that monounsaturated fats comprise the majority of your fat intake. Good sources include olive oil, canola oil, avocados, almonds, and hazelnuts. Table 2.6 outlines the types of fats contained in various oils.

Unfortunately what has gotten lost in some of this heart healthy advice are recommendations regarding the types of polyunsaturated fats that you should emphasize in your diet. Linoleic and alpha-linolenic essential fatty acids are both polyunsaturated

Being a Vegetarian Athlete

In recent years, many nutritionally aware endurance athletes have decreased their intake of proteins and meats high in saturated fat. Some have gone a step further and replaced animal proteins with plant proteins. Vegetarians are individuals who have consciously made the choice to completely exclude or include only specific animal foods in their diet, such as dairy products, eggs, or fish, and obtain a significant portion of their protein from plant foods. Whether these dietary modifications are for health, environmental, animal rights, or taste-related reasons, you need to pay as much attention to your vegetarian eating program as you do to your training program.

Vegetarianism is a term that actually incorporates a range of dietary exclusions. A plant-based vegetarian diet may refer to one of the following descriptions:

- **Semi- or near vegetarians**—eat small amounts of fish, poultry, eggs, and dairy, and avoid red meat
- **Pesco-vegetarians**—eat fish, dairy, and eggs
- **Lacto-ovo-vegetarians**—eat dairy foods and eggs
- **Ovo-vegetarians**—eat eggs
- **Vegans**—eat no animal foods

fats, but they differ greatly in how they affect our health. Linoleic acid is from a family of fats known as omega-6 fats, while alpha-linolenic is from the omega-3 family of fats. Two other omega-3 fats, docosahexanoic (DHA) and eicosapentaenoic (EPA), are abundant in fish oils such as salmon and tuna. The body can convert alpha-linolenic acid to DHA and EPA, though the conversion is inefficient.

DHA and EPA are of great interest to health experts. These fats, as well as alpha-linolenic acid, are needed to produce hormone-like compounds that can reduce

Depending on what type of vegetarian diet you follow, you need to carefully choose foods that provide specific nutrients in your diet. These nutrients include protein, iron, and zinc, and, particularly if you exclude dairy products, vitamin B_{12}, calcium, and vitamin D.

Throughout this book, the unique considerations of vegetarian athletes will be addressed in regard to specific nutrients. Of course any athlete can choose to include more plant sources of specific nutrients in their diet. Plant foods are filled with health promoting minerals. Vegetarians appear to have a lower risk of hypertension, certain cancers, and a decreased risk for developing heart disease and dia-

betes. A plant-based diet also supplies plenty of carbohydrates for replenishing body fuel stores after training. Whole grains, fruits, and vegetables as described are healthy sources of carbohydrates for any endurance athlete. Milk and yogurt, though sources of high quality protein, add nice amounts of carbohydrate to your diet as well.

However, vegetarian endurance athletes should pay close attention to their diet. Like a diet containing meat and other animal protein, a vegetarian diet can be well planned and support your training efforts, or it can be overly restrictive and ill-conceived and hamper your training efforts. ■

unnecessary blood clotting, boost immune function, and reduce inflammation. Conversely, excess linoleic acid can produce hormones that lead to inflammation, promote blood clotting, and promote constriction of arteries. Because linoleic and alpha-linolenic acid compete in the body for the same physiological pathway, it is best not to consume an excess of linoleic acid.

Keep in mind that both of these essential fats are good for you. What is desirable is to obtain the proper balance of the two essential fatty acids in your diet. However,

PERCENTAGES OF FATS IN VARIOUS OILS

Oil	% Saturated	% Polunsaturated	% Monounsaturated
Canola oil	6	32	62
Safflower oil	10	77	13
Sunflower oil	11	69	20
Corn oil	13	62	25
Olive oil	14	9	77
Soybean oil	15	61	24
Margarine (tub)*	17	34	24
Peanut oil	18	33	49
Cottonseed oil	27	54	19
Lard	41	12	47
Palm kernel oil	85	2	11
Coconut oil	92	2	6

Also contains some trans fatty acid

most North Americans consume an excess of linoleic fat and need to increase their intake of alpha-linolenic acid. Table 2.7 will guide you in choosing food sources of these fats. Try to emphasize fatty fish and use flax, soy, and canola oils. Olive oil supplies very little of these essential fats, but it is an excellent source of the healthy monounsaturated fat. Other good sources of alpha-linolenic acid include leafy green vegetables, walnuts, and flaxseed. Several foods are listed under both of these fat sources, as they are rich in both essential fatty acids. While scientists are still formulating specific recommendations, aim for a minimum of 2 grams of alpha-linolenic acid daily.

To emphasize the best fat choices, you can balance your intake in the following way:

- Consume fish and emphasize fatty fish like salmon, tuna, and mackerel two times weekly or more.
- Emphasize soy, walnut, flax, and canola oils and related products, and use olive oil as well.
- Include green leafy vegetables, walnuts, and ground flaxseed in your diet.
- Choose the leanest cuts of red meat possible.
- Limit fatty cheeses.

2.7

FOOD SOURCES OF ESSENTIAL FATTY ACIDS

FOODS RICH IN ALPHA-LINOLENIC ACID

Food	Alpha-linolenic Acid Content (g)
Flax oil, 1 Tbsp.	6.60
Flaxseed, ground, 1 Tbsp.	1.80
Soy nuts, roasted, 1/2 cup	1.80
Canola oil, 1 Tbsp.	1.60
Walnut oil, 1 Tbsp.	1.40
Soybean oil, 1 Tbsp.	1.00
Tofu, firm, 1/2 cup	0.70
Soy milk, 1 cup	0.40
Sardines, 2 oz.	0.28
Oat germ, 2 Tbsp.	0.20
Spinach, cooked, 1 cup	0.15
Kale, cooked, 1 cup	0.13
Almond butter, 2 Tbsp.	0.12
Wheat germ, 2 Tbsp.	0.10
Legumes, 1/2 cup	0.05

FOODS RICH IN LINOLEIC ACID

Food	Linoleic Acid Content (g)
Flaxseed, ground, 1 Tbsp.	11.0
Flax oil, 1 Tbsp.	10.1
Canola oil, 1 Tbsp.	9.2
Soy nuts, roasted, 1/2 cup	9.0
Soybean oil, 1 Tbsp.	7.8
Tofu, firm, 1/2 cup	7.0
Walnut oil, 1 Tbsp.	6.9
Soy milk, 1 cup	6.0
Legumes, 1/2 cup	5.4
Oat germ, 2 Tbsp.	4.5
Wheat germ, 2 Tbsp.	4.4
Spinach, cooked, 1 cup	3.8
Sardines, 2 oz.	3.0
Kale, cooked, 1 cup	0.8
Almond butter, 2 Tbsp.	0.5

- Emphasize poultry, beans, lentils, and soy protein in your diet.
- Control margarine intake, and choose products with liquid oil as the first ingredient.
- Avoid processed foods that contain partially hydrogenated oil and trans fat.

FIBER

Another good reason for choosing unprocessed carbohydrate foods is for the fiber they provide. This important nutrient has been linked to a reduced risk of heart disease, diabetes, and obesity. Fiber may also protect you from some forms of cancer. Fiber also can help prevent many conditions related to colon function including constipation, hemorrhoids, and diverticulosis.

Fiber is actually a class of compounds that can be divided into two main categories, water-soluble and water-insoluble fiber. Insoluble fiber is the most familiar form and is found in wheat bran, whole grain cereals, dried beans and peas, vegetables, and nuts. This type of fiber aids digestion and regulates colon function. Water-soluble fiber can help control blood glucose and blood cholesterol levels. Good sources of water-soluble fiber include whole oats, oat bran, some fruits, and dried beans. Fiber can also increase your feeling of fullness after consuming a meal, a useful tool for individuals trying to reduce their caloric intake and lose weight.

Nutrition experts recommend consuming between 20 to 30 grams of fiber daily. This amount can usually be reached by eating more than five servings of fruits and vegetables daily and several servings of whole grains. By consuming fiber from food sources you obtain a mix of fibers and other healthy nutrients that these foods provide, and the quantity of fiber you consume is consistent with your energy intake and not excessive.

Generally, excessive amounts of fiber and fiber supplements are not recommended. The result may be bloating and other unwanted gastrointestinal side effects. If you do need to increase the amount of fiber in your diet, do so gradually and drink plenty of water. Endurance athletes with very high caloric requirements may find that excessive fiber is too filling and replaces more concentrated and needed sources of calories. High fiber foods may also not be the best choices close to training and competition as they may cause intestinal discomfort with exercise. For the endurance athlete, fiber intake is not only about health but also about consuming the correct amounts at the safest times.

SUGAR

Sugar, the common name for sucrose, is the most prevalent simple carbohydrate in the North American diet. Nutritionists often refer to foods high in sugar as "empty calories" because of their low nutritional value. Sugar and other related substances such as fructose, glucose, and honey provide energy but not much else in the way of nutrients. Experts recommend that sugar comprise no more than 10 percent of our total energy intake, though many individuals consume greater than 20 percent of their total energy intake from sugar. Excess intake of refined sugar has been associated with high triglyceride levels and dental cavities. Excess sugar can also contribute to weight management problems.

Sugar is one of the major additives in processed foods and is often associated with a low fiber, high fat diet. Try to limit products in which sugar is the first ingredient on labels, and also look for labeling terms such as corn syrup, dextrose, and fructose that reflect a high sugar content. Naturally occurring sugars may work to satisfy a sweet tooth. Try sweet and dried fruits and jams to satisfy your sweet tooth. Of course, you are only human and may crave sugar at times. Just keep the sweet choices in perspective and have them as occasional treats in your daily training diet. Sugar, however, can play a much different role for the endurance athlete as it is a major component of many sports nutrition supplements designed for consumption during training and for recovery. They provide the required amounts of carbohydrates in easily digested forms.

PUTTING IT ALL TOGETHER

Choosing a wholesome diet is not about consuming the "perfect" diet. You achieve a balanced diet by making daily choices that should be viewed in the context of your whole day and even your entire week. Sometimes life gets in the way of making the

What Is Metabolic Syndrome?

Metabolic syndrome is a cluster of symptoms that may indicate an increased risk of developing diabetes and heart disease. One of the hallmarks of this syndrome is insulin resistance, which appears to have a strong genetic component, as well as being lifestyle- and diet-related. Two lifestyle risk factors for metabolic syndrome are being overweight and inactivity, usually not on the endurance athlete's top-ten list of concerns. However, some researchers have identified that possibly one-fourth of normal-weight individuals may have signs of metabolic syndrome. It is important to keep in mind that their data do not include physically active individuals, let alone endurance athletes. However, it is possible that because of your genetics, and possibly your blood work, you may want to learn more about this growing health concern.

Glucose intolerance and insulin resistance characterize metabolic syndrome. When the body is unable to respond to insulin, the pancreas produces more insulin until glucose can be carried out of the bloodstream and into the cells. When adequate insulin can no longer be produced, blood glucose levels stay elevated and the condition is known as diabetes. It is estimated that 60 million to 75 million Americans are insulin resistant.

Many individuals who are insulin resistant do not develop diabetes, but excess insulin can lead to other health concerns. It can cause a cluster of problems that raises the risk of heart disease. These problems include high triglyceride levels (a bad type of fat), low HDL cholesterol, hypertension, and body fat distributed on the upper body.

If you have blood work that indicates that metabolic syndrome may be a concern, rest assured that exercise is a very important part of treating this syndrome. Limiting your intake of saturated fat and emphasizing the monounsaturated fats, omega-3 polyunsaturated fats, and fiber are also recommended dietary guidelines that are consistent with your sports nutrition diet. But insulin resistant individuals are also advised to reduce their carbohydrate intake to less than 50 percent of total calories and to place an emphasis on low glycemic choices.

The message here for endurance athletes is to have your lipid profile checked, especially if you have a family history of diabetes and heart disease, then make the appropriate modifications in your fat intake. Avoid extremes in your carbohydrate intake that are beyond what you require for training, and emphasize lower glycemic choices when appropriate. However, you do not want to reduce your total carbohydrates to such a low level that you are not able to recover sufficiently from your training sessions and compromise your muscle glycogen stores. What is clear is that diets need to be individualized and that the best balance of carbohydrate and fat may not be the same for everyone. A qualified sports nutritionist who is familiar with your medical history can assist you in planning a sports diet that will not aggravate your health risk factors. Follow-up monitoring can fine-tune your diet as needed. ■

best choices, or practical issues determine what you will eat. Fitting in food around training schedules and work or school can often be challenging, and convenience will likely play a strong role in your food choices. Meals may often be consumed on the run when going from one commitment to the next. The key is to choose the most nutritious products whenever possible and to make the best choices available when convenience and practicality take precedence.

chapter 3

NUTRIENTS FOR OPTIMAL PERFORMANCE

A s an endurance athlete you are understandably interested in consuming an optimal amount of vitamins and minerals in your diet for both maximum performance and good health. You may find yourself questioning just how your training program may alter or increase your requirements of these important nutrients. And as an athlete, you also have a highly vested interest in keeping your immune system healthy so that illness does not put a halt to training. While athletes have long been advised by sports nutritionists to consume high quality foods for an optimal nutrient intake, advertising that targets active individuals seems to suggest that they need a daily vitamin and mineral supplement. Which is correct?

Of course choosing foods that provide you with adequate amounts of vitamins and minerals is necessary for optimal performance. Correcting any dietary inadequacies could even improve your performance. However, research has not conclusively proven that taking "extra" amounts of vitamins and minerals when no deficiency is present will enable you to train harder and longer. While all vitamins and minerals are important, it would benefit you to be aware of nutrients that are especially important to the endurance athlete.

VITAMIN BASICS

Vitamins consist of thirteen organic compounds found in small amounts in most foods. They play important roles in many physiological processes, many of which are greatly enhanced during exercise. Therefore it is wise to ensure that you have high levels of body reserves of these nutrients in order for these processes to function optimally. While it is true that inadequate intake of vitamins may result in deficiencies, whether or not it will adversely impact your performance depends upon the extent of that deficiency. Extreme deficiencies are not very commonplace in North America, and many

Optimal Health and Dietary Reference Intakes

With the release of guidelines by the National Academy of Sciences (NAS), the Recommended Daily Allowances (RDA) are finally reflecting goals consistent with the twenty-first century. Rather than merely preventing nutrient deficiencies, the new guidelines are set with the goal of optimizing health by reducing the risk of chronic diseases such as heart disease, cancer, and osteoporosis.

The new recommendations are officially known as Dietary Reference Intakes (DRI). Each updated nutrient has acquired a number of terms under the umbrella heading of DRI. The DRI values are provided in reports published over several years' time offering new guidelines on similarly grouped nutrients. Instead of a single category, the DRI include the four following classifications:

Recommended Daily Allowance (RDA): The amount of a nutrient that should decrease the risk of chronic disease for most healthy individuals in a spec-

dietary inadequacies can be corrected by making proper food choices. Athletes most likely to have problems with an inadequate vitamin intake are those following a restricted calorie diet for weight loss, athletes who have adopted an extreme or fad diet, and perhaps those on a very restrictive vegetarian diet. But overall, endurance athletes can greatly minimize their risk of vitamin deficiency by consuming a wide variety of nutrient dense foods and adequate calories to match their training needs.

Vitamins play a major role in catalyzing energy production reactions from body fuel stores. For instance, several B vitamins are essential to converting carbohydrates

ified age group and gender. It is based on estimating the average requirement plus an increase to account for individual variation. It is to serve as a goal for individuals only.

Adequate Intake (AI): Used when there is not enough scientific evidence to set an RDA. It is a recommended daily intake based on observed or experimentally determined approximations of nutrient intake by a group of healthy people. The AI can be used as a goal for individual intake when an RDA does not exist.

Estimated Average Requirement (EAR): A nutrient value estimated to meet the requirements of half the healthy individuals in a group. It is used to develop the RDA, assess adequacy of intakes, and plan diets for population groups.

Tolerable Upper Intake Level (UL): The highest level of a daily nutrient intake, from both food and supplements, which should not be exceeded or individuals are likely to experience adverse health affects. This is not a recommended amount. For most nutrients, the UL refers to the amount obtained from the total food intake, fortified foods, and supplements. ■

into energy for muscular contraction. Vitamins themselves do not directly provide energy, which must be obtained from consuming carbohydrates, protein, and fat. The vitamins B_{12} and B_6 and folic acid also play an important role in the development of red blood cells that deliver oxygen to the exercising muscles. Vitamins are also involved in tissue repair and protein synthesis. Several vitamins such as E and C are antioxidants that protect cells from potentially toxic "free radicals." Free radicals are unstable molecules produced by oxygen related reactions in the body and have been implicated in contributing to a number of diseases. Each vitamin is unique in the functions it performs in the body and in how it interacts with other dietary nutrients.

Vitamins are separated into two classifications, fat-soluble and water-soluble. Your body may contain large stores of the fat-soluble variety—A, D, E, and K. Deficiencies of these nutrients are rare, though excessive intakes may have toxic effects. The water-soluble variety—which include vitamin C and the eight B vitamins: thiamin (B_1), riboflavin (B_2), pyridoxine (B_6), niacin, B_{12}, folacin, biotin, and pantothenic acid—are not stored in your body in significant amounts. Harmful effects of excessive intakes of these water-soluble vitamins are not as likely, though there are exceptions. Appendix B provides a list of vitamins, their functions, and food sources.

IMPORTANT VITAMINS

B Vitamins

Due to their role in processing energy, B vitamins have received much attention from athletes. However, these vitamins are easily obtained from carbohydrate-rich foods such as breads and whole grains that are found in relatively high amounts in the endurance athlete's diet. Though these water-soluble vitamins are easily excreted, excesses of these nutrients can present a problem. Pyridoxine (vitamin B_6) in doses of more than one gram daily over several months may cause numbness and even paralysis. Symptoms have also been experienced with chronic doses as low as 200 milligrams. Excess niacin can block the release of free fatty acids, resulting in greater use of muscle glycogen and thereby depleting a limited energy source for endurance exercise, and large doses may actually reduce performance.

If you consume adequate servings of legumes, grains, fruit, vegetables, and nuts, you should have no difficulty meeting the requirements of most B vitamins. However, adequate intake of certain B vitamins may be an area of concern for the vegetarian athlete. Your vitamin B_{12} needs are easily met by consuming animal foods. So if you consume eggs and dairy foods, your intake should be fine. But the only plant foods that can be counted on for their B_{12} content are those that have been fortified with this vitamin. Some reliable fortified food sources are soy milk, soy burgers, and some breakfast cereals. Plant proteins such as tempeh and miso may not contain the active form of vitamin B_{12}. The human intestinal tract does make some vitamin B_{12} but this is generally not well absorbed. While requirements of this vitamin are relatively low, deficiencies can have serious implications and even lead to irreversible nerve damage. Vegans who do not regularly consume fortified foods should take a vitamin B_{12} supplement.

Another B vitamin that vegetarians should pay attention to is riboflavin, as milk, meat, and eggs are good sources. Some plant sources include brewer's yeast, wheat germ, soybeans, avocados, green leafy vegetables, and enriched bread and cereals. A well-planned vegetarian diet should be adequate in riboflavin.

Folacin

Folacin is a B vitamin that has deservedly received much increased attention from health professionals over the past several years. Folacin is the collective term for folate, folic acid, and other forms of the vitamin. Folate is the form found naturally in foods, and folic acid is the form of the vitamin found most often in your body and which is added to foods and supplements. Folic acid is actually absorbed twice as well as the folate that occurs naturally in foods.

Since January 1998, manufacturers have been required to add folic acid to all enriched products including flour, bread, rolls, grits, corn meal, rice, pasta, and noodles. There is good reason for this fortification. Obtaining enough folic acid in the early weeks of pregnancy can significantly reduce the risk of neural tube defects such as spina bifida in newborns. Prior to fortification, most Americans consumed only about 200 micrograms of folic acid daily, falling short of the recommended 400 micrograms. Fortification will prevent half of all neural tube defects. But this fortification may not only benefit pregnant women and newborns.

Evidence is building that folic acid may reduce the risk of heart disease, stroke, and certain cancers. Folic acid helps reduce blood levels of the amino acid homocysteine. High levels of homocysteine appear to be a strong predictor of heart disease and stroke. Keeping homocysteine low also requires adequate intake of the vitamins B_6 and B_{12}. Thirty percent of all older Americans don't produce enough stomach acid to absorb the B_{12} found in foods. Synthetic B_{12}, however, doesn't have this stomach acid dependency. Connections between folic acid and the prevention of cervical cancer and colorectal cancer, through prevention of damage to DNA, have also been suggested.

3.1

FOLATE-RICH FOODS

Food	Folate Content (mcg)
Lentils, cooked, 1 cup	358
Yeast, brewer's, 1 Tbsp.	312
Liver, beef, 3 oz.	285
Garbanzo beans, cooked, 1 cup	282
Kidney beans, cooked, 1 cup	229
Turnip greens, cooked, 1 cup	171
Asparagus, boiled, 6 spears	131
Beans, white, baked, 1 cup	122
Orange juice, 1 cup	110
Spinach, raw, chopped, 1 cup	108
Mustard greens, cooked, 1 cup	103
Broccoli, cooked, 1 cup	78
Romaine lettuce, 1 cup	76
Endive, 1 cup	72
Wheat germ, raw, 1/4 cup	70

Many researchers suggest that individuals over the age of 50 take a supplement providing the RDA (high doses are not advised) of folic acid, B_{12}, and B_6. Older individuals are also more likely to take medications that interfere with folic acid absorption. Of course, every active individual should increase the intake of folate rich foods. See Table 3.1 for a list of folate rich foods.

Antioxidant Nutrients

Vitamin C

Another water-soluble vitamin of interest to and heavily marketed to athletes is vitamin C. Several important functions of this vitamin impact athletes. It is necessary for the formation of connective tissue and scar tissue, as well as certain hormones and neurotransmitters that are secreted during exercise. Vitamin C plays a role in iron absorption and in the formation of red blood cells. This vitamin is also strongly promoted because of its role as a powerful antioxidant. Symptoms of vitamin C deficiency could impair athletic performance.

Despite being a water-soluble vitamin that is easily excreted, the human body actually has a pool of vitamin C ranging from 1.5 to 3.0 grams. Serious vitamin C deficiencies are rare because fresh or frozen fruits and vegetables are so abundant in our food supply. Though vitamin C is readily available from food, athletes often consume vitamin C supplements. Correcting a deficiency clearly improves performance, but research does not demonstrate that vitamin C supplements enhance performance when a vitamin C deficiency is not present.

On the other hand, because exercise places stress on the body, moderate amounts of vitamin C above the RDA of 75–90 milligrams may be appropriate for athletes. Some scientists have recommended 200–300 milligrams daily. Research indicates that 200 milligrams daily of vitamin C leads to full saturation of plasma and white blood cells, which supports optimal immune function. Vitamin C supplements may also reduce the symptoms and duration of upper respiratory tract infections often seen after strenuous physical efforts. However, most studies have

3.2
VITAMIN C CONTENT OF FOOD

Food	Vitamin C (mg)
Pepper, green, 1 large	130
Orange juice, 1 cup	124
Cranberry juice, 1 cup	108
Grapefruit juice, 1 cup	94
Broccoli, cooked, 2/3 cup	90
Brussels sprouts, cooked, 7	85
Strawberries, raw, 1 cup	85
Orange, navel, 1	80
Kiwifruit, 1 medium	75
Cantaloupe, pieces, 1 cup	70
Cauliflower, cooked, 1 cup	65

not found that vitamin C supplementation prevents colds. A diet rich in fruits and vegetables provides ample amounts of vitamin C and other healthful substances found in those foods. Table 3.2 lists the vitamin C content of some top sources of this nutrient.

You can consider up to a 500-gram dose of vitamin C prior to an ultraendurance event in order to protect your immune system. Avoid excessive intakes of 1,000–3,000 milligrams daily, which can cause side effects such as diarrhea and kidney stones.

Vitamin E

Vitamin E also receives much attention from athletes because of its major role as an antioxidant. This vitamin prevents the oxidation of unsaturated fatty acids in cell membranes and protects the cell from damage. Vitamin E is widely distributed in foods and stored in the body, so vitamin E deficiencies are rare. The current RDI is 22 International Units (IU). Polyunsaturated oils such as soybean, corn, and safflower are the most common sources of vitamin E. Other good sources are fortified grain products and wheat germ.

Experiments on vitamin E supplementation at altitude have produced some interesting results, but more research is required, especially to determine if there are any real performance benefits. Vitamin E may also be beneficial to athletes training in high-pollution areas due to its antioxidant effects. Though no performance benefits have been established, vitamin E supplements may be recommended for possible prevention of chronic diseases, especially heart disease. Some researchers currently feel that a daily supplement dose of 100–400 IU is safe and appropriate.

Persons with a bleeding disorder or on anticoagulant medication or statin medications designed to lower elevated blood lipids should be cautious and first check with their physician before taking vitamin E. If you do take a vitamin E supplement, choose one that provides the natural source of the vitamin. See Table 3.3 for good sources of vitamin E.

3.3

VITAMIN E CONTENT OF FOODS

Food	Portion	Vitamin E (IU)
Wheat germ oil	1 Tbsp.	25
Sunflower seeds	1 oz.	21
Almonds	1 oz.	11
Sunflower oil	1 Tbsp.	10
Wheat germ	1 oz.	5
Brown rice	1 cup	3
Margarine, soft	1 Tbsp.	3
Mayonnaise	1 Tbsp.	3
Mango	1 medium	3
Asparagus	4 spears	2

Carotenoids

Beta-carotene is just one of 600 carotenoid pigments that give fruits and vegetables their yellow, orange, and red colors. Carotenoids are also abundant in green vegetables. While carotenoids are not vitamins, many act as antioxidants and also protect cells from free radicals.

Carotenoids most commonly found in blood and tissues are alpha-carotene, beta-carotene, beta-cryptoxanthin, lutein, lycopene, and zeaxanthin. Only alpha-carotene, beta-carotene and beta-cryptoxanthin can be converted to vitamin A in the body. Research is just beginning to determine how specific carotenoids can boost immunity and protect the heart and eyes from chronic disease.

To obtain a variety of carotenoids in your diet, aim for at least five servings combined of fruits and vegetables daily, focusing mainly on yellow-orange, red, or dark green choices. You can easily obtain ample amounts in your diet. See Table 3.4 for good sources of carotenoids.

Taking a supplement with carotenoids requires some caution, particularly in the case of beta-carotene supplements, which were found to increase cancer in smokers. It is advised not to supplement, but stay under 3 milligrams daily if you do take a supplement. In addition, carotenoids interact with one another. Supplementing with one carotenoid may impair the absorption of others. Carotenoids are converted to vitamin A as the body requires. But vitamin A supplements can be highly toxic at greater than the daily RDA of 5,000 IU. Besides, foods high in carotenoids may provide health-promoting substances not found in supplements. It's quite possible that these protective nutrients work best when they are packaged together, as in food.

3.4

GOOD SOURCES OF CAROTENOIDS

FOODS HIGH IN CAROTENOIDS

(Including alpha-carotene, beta-carotene, beta-cryptoxanthin, lutein, zeaxanthin, lycopene)

Food	Portion
Apricot, dried	6 halves
Broccoli, cooked	1/2 cup
Cantaloupe, chunks	1 cup
Carrot, raw	1 medium
Collard greens, cooked	1/2 cup
Grapefruit	1/2 medium
Kale, cooked	1/2 cup
Mango	1 medium
Mustard greens, cooked	1/2 cup
Orange	1 medium
Papaya	1/2 medium
Pepper, red	1/2 raw
Pumpkin, cooked or canned	1/2 cup
Spinach, raw	1/2 cup
Sweet potato, mashed	1/2 cup
Tangerine	1 medium
Tomato sauce	1/2 cup

Phytochemicals

While vitamin A can be formed from some carotenoids, this group of nutrients is actually one of many that fall under the broader classification of phytochemicals. Many important disease-fighting properties have been attributed to these plant chemicals. Unlike vitamins and minerals, phytochemicals are not nutrients. Most phytochemicals are found in carbohydrate-containing foods such as fruits, vegetables, and grains. Some phytochemicals you may have heard about include: allylic sulfides found in garlic, flavonoids found in citrus fruits, genistein found in soybeans, indoles in broccoli and cauliflower, and phytoestrogens in soy products, to name a few. To take advantage of these phytochemicals, eat plenty of fruits and vegetables, dried peas and beans, and soy products. In the future, probably even more phyto-chemicals will be discovered.

MINERAL BASICS

Like vitamins, minerals are involved in energy metabolism and also play important roles in building body tissue, in muscle contraction and oxygen transport, in main-taining acid-base balance of the blood, and in regulating normal heart rhythm. Minerals are obtained in our diet from the water we drink and are found in both plant and animal foods. Training-induced mineral losses can occur through urine, sweat, and gastrointestinal losses.

There are twenty-five essential minerals, all with their own unique functions. Two very important minerals to the endurance athlete are calcium, which plays an essential role in maintaining healthy bone structure, and iron, which plays a crucial role in oxygen transport.

Important Minerals

Calcium

Calcium is the most abundant mineral in the body. Ninety-eight percent of calcium is found in bone, a dynamic tissue that is constantly being broken down and rebuilt. The remaining 2 percent of calcium in your body is in your teeth and cir-culates in your bloodstream.

This circulating calcium has a significant effect on metabolism and physiological functions. It is involved in all types of muscle contraction, including the heart muscle, skeletal muscle, and smooth muscle found in blood vessels. By activating a number of enzymes, calcium also plays a role in both the synthesis and breakdown of muscle and liver glycogen. Calcium is also involved in nerve impulse transmission, blood clotting, and secretion of hormones. These physiological functions of calcium take precedence over formation of bone tissue. If the diet is low in calcium, calcium can be pulled from the bone for these functions.

Calcium deficiency can develop from inadequate intake or increased calcium excretion. Strenuous exercise increases sweat loss of calcium. One of the major health concerns associated with inadequate intake of calcium is osteoporosis, a disorder in which bone mass decreases and susceptibility to fracture increases. Optimal bone building takes place until age 25, but you can continue to build some bone until 35 years of age. After this age your efforts should focus on maintaining your current level of bone mass.

Hormonal status, more specifically estrogen loss, also contributes significantly to the development of osteoporosis, making women more susceptible to this disease after menopause occurs, though men can also develop osteoporosis. Hormonal status in younger female athletes also plays an important role in bone health. Extra calcium is recommended for female athletes with absent or irregular menstruation and for post-menopausal athletes. Weight-bearing exercise such as running and weight training enhances calcium skeletal absorption, increases bone mass, and can help prevent bone loss at any age. Calcium recommendations for various ages are provided in Table 3.5. Vitamin D recommendations are also provided, as this vitamin is essential for adequate calcium absorption. As we age, our bodies become less efficient at converting sunlight to vitamin D.

3.5

CALCIUM AND VITAMIN D REQUIREMENTS

Age	Calcium	Vitamin D
19–50	1,000 mg	200 IU
51–70	1,200 mg (on hormone replacement therapy [HRT]) 1,500 mg (not on HRT)	400 IU
Over 70	1,200 mg (on HRT) 1,500 mg (not on HRT)	600 IU

3.6

FOOD SOURCES OF CALCIUM

GREAT SOURCES 300 mgs serving	GOOD SOURCES 200 mgs serving	FAIR SOURCES 100 mgs serving
1% Milk, 8 oz.	Bok choy, fresh, 1 cup	Cottage cheese, 1%, 1 cup
Blackstrap molasses, 2 Tbsp.	Brick cheese, 1 oz.	Figs, dried or fresh, 5 medium
Collard greens, cooked, 1 cup	Broccoli, cooked, 1 cup	Frozen yogurt, 1/2 cup
Mackerel, canned, 3 oz.	Cheddar cheese, 1 oz.	Lobster, cooked, 6 oz.
Orange juice, calcium fortified, 1 cup	Colby cheese, 1 oz.	Navy beans, cooked, 1 cup
Rhubarb, cooked, 1 cup	Edam cheese, 1 oz.	Orange, 1 large
Salmon, canned, w/bones, 3 oz.	Instant breakfast, 1 packet	Parmesan, 1 1/2 Tbsp.
Sardines, canned, w/bones, 3 oz.	Kale, cooked, 1 cup	Pinto beans, 1 cup
Skim milk, 8 oz.	Mozzarella cheese, 1 oz.	Pudding, 1/2 cup
Swiss cheese, 1 oz.	Mustard greens, cooked, 1 cup	Shrimp, cooked, 6 oz.
Yogurt, 6–8 oz.	Sesame seeds, 2 Tbsp.	Skim milk, dry, 1 Tbsp.
	Soybeans, cooked, 1 cup	Swiss chard, cooked, 1 cup
	Turnip greens, cooked, 1 cup	Tempeh, cooked, 1 cup
		Tofu, 1/2 cup

Dairy products are very concentrated sources of calcium and for most individuals provide about three-fourths of their total calcium intake. Vegan athletes and athletes who do not have a high intake of dairy products need to focus on alternative plant sources of calcium intake and increase their intake of calcium fortified foods. Try to choose low fat options as much as possible. Some good plant sources of calcium include dark leafy greens, broccoli, bok choy, dried beans, and dried figs. Some good fortified sources (check labels) are soy and rice milk, orange juice, cereals, tofu processed with calcium sulfate, and various energy bars. Look for products marked as "high" or "rich in" or an "excellent" source of calcium. They contain more than 200 milligrams per serving. Some good calcium sources are listed in Table 3.6. Individuals who are lactose intolerant can buy specially formulated lactose-free milks, or take lactase supplement enzymes before consuming milk products. Yogurt and cheese have lower lactose levels than milk and may be well tolerated. You may also be able to tolerate small amounts of lactose-containing foods.

A well-balanced training diet should provide many of the essential nutrients needed to build and maintain healthy bones. However, a calcium supplement may also be indicated if your food intake is not adequate. If you do take a calcium supplement, find one that provides more than 500 milligrams per pill and take one pill at a time. Amounts greater than 500–600 milligrams will not be fully absorbed. Calcium carbonate should be taken with meals to increase absorption, while the calcium citrate form can be taken at any time. Avoid calcium made from oyster shells, bone meal, or dolomite as it may contain lead.

Good food sources of vitamin D are relatively limited. They include fatty fish and egg yolks. Fortified sources include milk, soy milk, butter, margarine, and cereals. Fortunately, endurance athletes spend a considerable amount of time outdoors, and your body can make enough vitamin D when your skin is exposed to sunlight. However, sun exposure may not be adequate from October to April in the northern parts of the U.S. and in Canada. Our ability to make vitamin D from sunlight also decreases as we age. Older athletes, those living in northern climates, and vegetarians may want to consider taking a vitamin D supplement. Vitamin D is often conveniently combined with calcium in supplement form and can also be obtained from a multivitamin.

There are other nutrients that are also an important part of building healthy bones. These nutrients are briefly described below:

Vitamin C—Plays a role in collagen production, which helps hold bone together. A diet with plenty of fresh fruits and vegetables provides ample amounts.

Vitamin K—Activates osteocalcin, which is needed for optimal bone strength. Good sources are dark leafy green vegetables.

Magnesium—Another important mineral for bone formation. Good sources are almonds, bananas, avocados, dried beans, lentils, nuts, tofu, wheat germ, and whole grains.

In contrast, some dietary factors are actually harmful to calcium absorption. Excess sodium, protein, and caffeine increase calcium excretion. Alcohol can also be damaging to bone cells. Try not to consume excessive amounts of caffeine. Keep your protein intake at an appropriate level for training, but do not consume excessive and unneeded amounts from supplements.

Obtaining adequate calcium in your diet takes planning. Below are some tips for maximizing your calcium intake:

- Have a breakfast every day that includes high calcium milk, yogurt, or calcium fortified soy product.
- Plan a high calcium food into three meals or snacks daily.
- Prepare or order low fat milk and soy milk smoothies whenever possible.
- Make stir-fried vegetables for dinners that include one of the following: bok choy, kale, broccoli, or leafy greens.
- Add reduced fat cheeses to sandwiches.
- Drink a glass of calcium fortified orange juice on a regular basis.
- Buy tofu high in calcium for stir-fries and other recipes.

Iron

Many athletes are aware of the important roles that iron plays in exercise metabolism. Hemoglobin transports oxygen in the blood, and myoglobin transports oxygen in the muscle. Both of these oxygen-carrying molecules require iron for optimal formation. Many muscle enzymes involved in metabolism require iron. Other iron compounds facilitate oxygen use at the cellular level. The body storage form of iron, ferritin, is used as an indicator of iron stores, as are transferrin and hemoglobin. About 70 percent of the iron in your body is involved in oxygen transport, while the other 30 percent is stored in the body. It makes sense that poor iron status could impair these functions and exercise performance. This has been demonstrated when an athlete has iron deficiency that has progressed to anemia. Anemia causes fatigue and intolerance to exercise.

Iron deficiency is the most common nutrient deficiency in the United States. It is estimated that 22 to 25 percent of female athletes are iron deficient, with 6 percent having full-blown anemia. When iron stores are low, total hemoglobin drops, and the muscles do not receive as much oxygen. Normal hemoglobin levels for males are 14–16 grams per deciliter (gm/dl), with anemia classified as less than 13 gm/dl. The normal range for women is 12–14 gm/dl, with anemia diagnosed at less than 12 gm/dl. Blood work can be interpreted to determine if you have early iron deficiency or full iron deficiency anemia. However, endurance training can affect your blood measurements of iron. Training produces an increased blood volume, which dilutes hemoglobin, making it appear low in some athletes when iron stores are adequate. This increased blood volume often occurs at the start of a training program and has no harmful effect on performance. In fact this increased blood volume means that your heart can pump more blood to your working muscles, enhancing oxygen delivery.

Data clearly indicates that true iron deficiency anemia will impair exercise performance. While there is less data regarding the performance effects of a low ferritin level, athletes may experience symptoms of fatigue and poor recovery with this condition. Of course, it makes sense to treat low ferritin levels so that full-blown iron deficiency anemia does not develop and to improve any reoccurring symptoms. Your blood work should be monitored by a physician and treated as appropriate.

Inadequate dietary intake of iron is the most common cause of iron deficiency or anemia. Women with heavy menstrual blood loss may also experience iron deficiency. Strenuous exercise can also increase iron sweat loss, precipitate gastrointestinal bleeding, and decrease iron absorption. Strenuous training may also accelerate red blood cell destruction from mechanical trauma, such as during running. Training at altitude can also place you at risk for developing iron deficiency. Development of iron deficiency is also associated with low calorie diets, vegetarian diets, very high carbohydrate diets containing only small amounts of animal protein, and various fad and unbalanced diets.

Iron is obtained from food in two forms. Heme iron is found in animal foods—good sources are lean meat and dark poultry. About 10 to 30 percent of heme iron is absorbed from the intestines. Non-heme iron is found in plant foods—dried peas and beans, whole grain products, apricots, and raisins are good sources. About 2 to 10 percent of non-heme iron is absorbed. Non-heme iron absorption is compromised by the phytates that are found in many vegetables and whole grains.

Consuming meats and plant iron sources together can enhance iron absorption from plant foods. Small amounts of red meat in bean chili, spinach with chicken, and turkey with lentil soup combine heme and non-heme iron. Vitamin C-containing foods also enhance plant iron absorption. Try having orange juice or strawberries with fortified cereal. Table 3.7 lists good sources of iron.

3.7

IRON CONTENT OF SELECTED FOODS

Sources of Heme Iron	
Liver, beef, cooked, 3 oz.	6.0 mg
Beef, cooked, 3 oz.	3.5 mg
Pork, cooked, 3 oz.	3.4 mg
Shrimp, cooked, 3 oz.	2.6 mg
Turkey, dark, cooked, 3 oz.	2.0 mg
Chicken, breast, cooked, 3 oz.	1.0 mg
Tuna, light, 3 oz.	1.0 mg
Flounder, sole, salmon, 3 oz.	1.0 mg

Sources of Plant Iron	
Cereal, iron-fortified	2–18 mg
Cream of wheat, 3/4 cup	9.0 mg
Lentils, 1 cup	6.0 mg
Instant breakfast, 1 envelope	4.5 mg
Kidney beans, canned, 1 cup	3.2 mg
Baked potato, with skin, 1	3.0 mg
Prune juice, 8 oz.	3.0 mg
Wheat germ, 1/4 cup	2.6 mg
Apricots, dried, 10 halves	1.7 mg
Spaghetti, enriched, cooked, 1/2 cup	1.4 mg
Bread, enriched, 1 slice	1.0 mg

To boost iron intake you can:

- Incorporate lean meat regularly into your diet. Have small amounts several times weekly.

- Try adding small amounts of red meats to your favorite recipes like stir-fry, soups, pasta sauces, and casseroles.

- Mix heme-iron foods with non-heme choices, such as bean chili with dark turkey meat.

- Incorporate iron fortified cereals into your diet.

- Increase fish and shellfish in your diet.

- Increase your intake of plant irons such as whole grain cereals, legumes, and green leafy vegetables. Eat them with a vitamin C-containing food.

Endurance athletes training at altitude and female endurance athletes may want to supplement with the RDA of iron. Many multivitamins contain this amount of iron so check labels. You should also have your hemoglobin, hematocrit, and ferritin stores monitored regularly. Taking excess iron from supplements, however, does carry some risk.

Iron and Zinc Supplements

Zinc is another important mineral for endurance athletes. An adequate amount of zinc keeps your immune system strong and promotes healing of wounds and injuries. Zinc is also a component of several enzymes involved in energy metabolism and is involved in protein synthesis. Good sources of zinc include red meat, turkey, milk, yogurt, and seafood—especially oysters. The zinc from animal foods is better absorbed than that found in plant foods. Plant sources of zinc include garbanzo beans, lentils, lima beans, brown rice, and wheat germ.

It is important that you do not self-diagnose low iron stores, but rather have your blood work evaluated by a physician. If you take a supplement providing greater than 100 percent of the RDA for iron and zinc, your hemoglobin, hematocrit, and ferritin should be monitored regularly. Higher doses of iron, even as little as 25 milligrams, can inhibit absorption of zinc and another mineral, copper. Oversupplementing with zinc can also interfere with absorption of other minerals. Excess iron supplementation may also adversely affect individuals who have a genetic predisposition to iron overload. Iron overload, a condition known as hemochromatosis, is a genetic disorder that affects one in every 200 people. This condition can result in excess iron deposits in the heart, liver, joints, and various body tissues, with the potential for damaging these tissues. High levels of iron supplements can also lead to gastrointestinal intolerance and constipation. Vegetarians can consider a supplement that provides 100 percent of the Daily Values for iron and other trace minerals such as zinc and copper to ensure that they obtain adequate amounts of these nutrients.

Multivitamin Mineral Supplements

Endurance athletes have the distinct advantage of being able to eat more than their sedentary counterparts. With a focus on quality food choices, this generally means a diet filled with variety and nutrients. While a multivitamin mineral supplement does guarantee that you will obtain all the Daily Values for vitamins and minerals, it is not the same as eating food. Nutrients from foods tend to be optimally absorbed and will provide you with all the phytochemicals, undiscovered or otherwise, that are not in your supplement. However, a broad-range, reasonable dose supplement may just be that little extra insurance that athletes who care about their health often seek. However, there are some active individuals who may want to seriously consider taking a vitamin and mineral supplement. This would be the case for athletes who consume fewer than 1,500 calories daily; have food allergies that restrict a significant number of choices from one food group; travel frequently; have disordered eating and erratic diets; are vegans or vegetarians who may need additional vitamin D, zinc, iron, B_{12} and riboflavin; are picky eaters who may restrict many foods; are at risk for osteoporosis; or are pregnant or planning a pregnancy.

If you decide to take a multivitamin mineral supplement, try to stick to the following guidelines:

- Choose a broad-range, balanced supplement of vitamins and minerals that provides 100 percent of the Daily Values (DV). These doses are known to be safe.
- Avoid supplements that contain an excess of minerals or any one mineral, as these nutrients compete with one another for absorption.
- Choose a supplement with the USP stamp of approval on the label to guarantee that it dissolves properly in your body.
- Choose a supplement in which the majority of vitamin A is actually beta-carotene, the precursor to vitamin A.
- A blend of natural and synthetic supplements is fine.
- Calcium and magnesium may need to be purchased separately as they are too bulky for a regular multivitamin pill.

- If you take antioxidant supplements, keep doses to 100 to 400 IU vitamin E and 250 milligrams vitamin C.
- Take your multivitamin with a meal or snack and plenty of water.

Antioxidant supplements are strongly marketed to athletes, but it is actually diets abundant in foods that contain antioxidant nutrients that have been shown to prevent cancer and other diseases. So don't discount the importance of increasing food sources of these nutrients. You may also wonder if training increases the effects of free radicals or if athletes learn to cope with these negative byproducts. Probably both situations occur. It is impossible to directly measure free-radical production in humans. Free radical byproducts do increase with exercise, but trained athletes may dispose of them more effectively.

Moderate doses of vitamin C, beta-carotene, and other carotenoids are easily obtained with educated food choices. However, one nutrient that may be difficult to obtain at antioxidant levels on a diet under 30-percent fat is vitamin E. Good sources are high in fat, and you would need to consume large amounts of them to reach even the low antioxidant dose of 100 IU. Researchers still need to determine the optimal doses of antioxidant supplements needed for preventing heart disease and cancer.

If you do supplement, do so wisely. A multivitamin and mineral supplement providing 100 percent of the DV should be safe, though not always necessary. But keep in mind that the hazards of vitamin and mineral overdosing are real and can be subtle. If you take a supplement, understand the good reasons for taking it, consume appropriate doses, and discontinue its use when it is no longer needed.

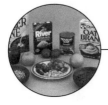

TRAINING NUTRITION

Fine-tuning Your Diet for Top Performance

A good training diet is built upon a solid foundation of wholesome food choices, but it takes more than good foods to support you in performing your best. Endurance training places high energy demands on your body, and optimal recovery is essential for quality training. Not only do your food choices matter, but how you portion and time your foods and fluids before, during, and after exercise can also positively impact your training efforts. Maximizing the amount of fuel you have available while training and replenishing your fuel stores for the next training session requires that you fine-tune your nutrition program until it becomes a routine part of your daily life. Fine-tuning your nutrition practices during training will also identify the nutrition techniques that work best for you during competition. To bring all this important information together, a very practical chapter will provide you with some concrete strategies for conveniently planning and consuming an optimal training diet. Guidelines for food shopping and eating out are provided, with sample menus.

Part II also outlines the safest and most effective nutrition strategies available to achieve an appropriate body composition so that you can be a lean and strong endurance athlete. And because sports nutrition supplements are so integral to your training, they will be reviewed along with the science behind the claims for the numerous ergogenic aids marketed to endurance athletes.

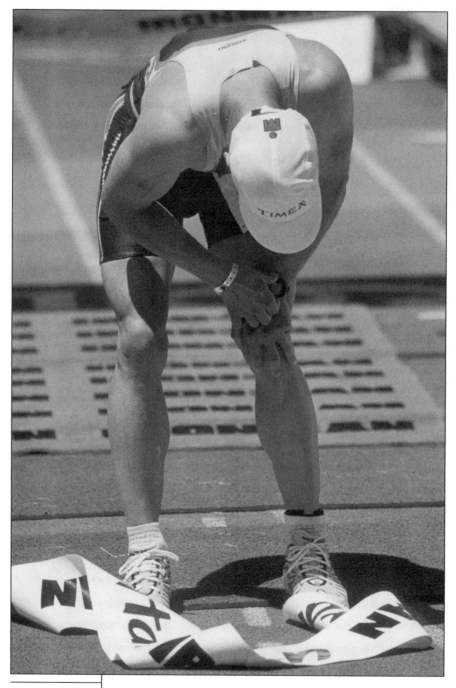

TOM MORAN PHOTO

chapter *4*

EATING FOR OPTIMAL RECOVERY

A Balance of Supply and Demand

There are several essential nutrition practices that transform a healthy, well-balanced diet into a scientifically sound, cutting-edge sports nutrition plan designed to support your training and recovery. These practices include:

- Consuming enough energy or calories.
- Consuming enough grams of carbohydrates to match that day's training and to prepare for the next training session.
- Timing your intake of carbohydrates to expedite the process of muscle glycogen resynthesis.
- Eating adequate amounts of protein for recovery, muscle tissue repair, and maintaining a strong immune system.
- Consuming fat to balance out the diet, provide essential fatty acids, and replenish muscle triglyceride levels.
- Consuming adequate amounts of fluid and electrolytes, particularly sodium for optimal recovery.
- Practicing immediate post-exercise nutrition recovery guidelines.

Most importantly, as an endurance athlete you must consume the right amount of energy or calories. Endurance training can be tough and tiring, and eating enough food is essential to completing longer exercise bouts at the intensities outlined in your program. The intensity and duration of your training also controls the types of fuel your body demands and best utilizes for energy. Because of their integral role in fueling endurance exercise and the limitations of your body's fuel stores, carbohydrates are the foundation of your training diet, with protein and fat also playing important supporting roles. Recovery is the process of eating properly, which provides you with the fuel to go from one training session to the next with the energy required. This process may need to take place in twenty-four hours, or perhaps even twelve, eight, or four hours, depending on your training schedule. Begin by choosing quality foods for your sports diet as outlined in Part I to lay the foundation for your diet. Once a solid foundation of good nutrition choices is established, consuming the optimal fuel for recovery and endurance training and putting in your best performance comes down to consuming these foods in the right amounts at the right times.

STORED FUEL: YOUR ENERGY SOURCE

Your muscles contain three different power systems that supply your body with energy for training. But ultimately, only one source of fuel can be used for muscle contraction, adenosine triphosphate (ATP). You are constantly using ATP for both daily living and training, whether to simply breathe, go to work, pump up your bicycle tires with air, or run ten miles. ATP is a high-energy chemical compound found in all muscle cells. When ATP is broken down, the energy released is used for muscle contraction. Because your muscles contain only a small amount of ATP, it must be steadily recharged for training to continue. The rate at which ATP is recharged in your body must meet the demands of the exercise you are performing. Lower intensity exercise requires a steady supply of ATP, while higher intensity exercise requires a more rapid supply of ATP. There are three energy systems that fuel your muscles:

ATP-CP or phosphagen system

Anaerobic glycolysis or lactic acid system

Aerobic system, both glycolytic (carbohydrate) and lipolytic (fat)

Because your body stores ATP in only small amounts, you require plenty of stored energy to recharge ATP and keep the energy flowing while you train. Body stores of carbohydrates, protein, and fat release varying amounts of ATP at varying rates when they are burned for fuel. Carbohydrates are stored in limited amounts in your blood as glucose and in your muscles and liver as glycogen. Blood glucose is your brain's sole source of energy at rest and during exercise. A steady supply of blood glucose keeps you focused while you negotiate a tricky turn on your bike or perfect your swim technique.

However, your blood glucose levels can quickly run low to meet the energy demands of endurance training. When this occurs, the liver breaks down its supply of glycogen into glucose and releases it directly into the bloodstream to maintain your blood glucose levels. A well-fed liver can store up to 400 calories of glycogen. But liver glycogen is a relatively short-lived fuel supply that fills up and empties depending on the timing and composition of your last meal. Depending on what you ate and how much, liver glycogen stores generally last from three to five hours. You have likely experienced some of the symptoms that come with low blood glucose levels when you have not eaten for several hours. This hunger, which signals the need for fuel, can occur three hours after breakfast, in the afternoon, before an evening training session, or any time that your liver stores run low.

Clearly your liver glycogen and blood glucose levels are a relatively limited supply of fuel. In fact, they can both become depleted relatively quickly during endurance training. As will be discussed in Chapter 5, endurance athletes can offset these losses by eating properly before training and competition and by consuming carbohydrates during exercise.

In contrast to your liver glycogen stores, your muscle glycogen is a much larger storage supply of energy, providing anywhere from 1,400 to 1,800 calories depending on your body weight and the makeup of your diet. When you train at any intensity from easy to hard, this glycogen is converted to glucose and used by the muscle fibers for energy. However, when your muscle glycogen stores run low, as can occur during steady long runs and bike rides or during hard interval training sessions, your muscles can also utilize the glucose in your bloodstream for fuel. Because you are an endurance athlete, you are constantly using your glycogen stores while training at most intensity levels and must replenish them by consuming adequate amounts of carbohydrates in your diet. How many carbohydrates you actually need, or the rate at which you burn carbohydrates (fast or slow), depends on how hard and how long you train that day.

Endurance athletes benefit greatly from ensuring that their muscle glycogen stores are refueled after training sessions that significantly deplete these stores. Several days of successive training without adequate glycogen replacement could ultimately result in poor energy levels and poor training.

Table 4.1 clearly outlines that your body's supply of carbohydrates is relatively limited. These carbohydrate stores provide enough fuel for only about ninety minutes to two hours of training, and even less during very high intensity exercise. You have probably experienced the symptoms of low body carbohydrate stores during one training session or another. When your blood glucose levels hit bottom you "bonk," and you may feel dizzy and unable to focus and concentrate. Most endurance athletes clearly remember the first time they bonked during exercise. You may have had to stop exercise altogether or slow down considerably while consuming carbohydrates to get your blood glucose levels back up. Bonking is not convenient at any time during exercise and can even be unsafe when riding in a pack or running with a group. You have probably also experienced muscle glycogen depletion and "hit the wall" and found putting one foot in front of the other difficult. Endurance athletes can simply avoid these energy draining training experiences by starting exercise properly fueled and by consuming enough carbohydrates during exercise to offset body fuel losses. More information on the proper nutrition techniques to practice while training will be covered in Chapter 5.

A quick look at Table 4.1 demonstrates that fat is the body's greatest supply of energy even in the leanest athletes, providing more than 80,000 stored calories.

During exercise, your muscles easily access the fat stored within your muscle cells, known as intramuscular triglycerides. Just like your muscle glycogen stores, intramuscular triglycerides must be replenished after training. Depending on the intensity and duration of the training session, you will also tap into the fat stored in adipose tissue and convert it to fatty acids that are transported to your muscles. It is these more visible body fat stores that provide a relatively unlimited supply of fat for fuel and that are often a focus of the weight management efforts of some endurance athletes.

Muscle protein stores can also potentially supply several thousand calories of energy. However, breaking down your muscle protein for fuel is not ideal for either your recovery or health. Muscle tissue maintains strength, and constant excess breakdown of this tissue places undue stress upon your body and your immune system. It is important to appreciate that during long rides, runs, and ski sessions, some of the amino acids that make up protein in the muscle can be converted to glucose for fuel. While a small percentage of your fuel during training can be safely derived from protein (about 5 percent), percentages reaching 15 percent are possible but not ideal.

Preventing muscle tissue breakdown can best be accomplished by maintaining optimal carbohydrate consumption during ultraendurance sessions. This outside source of glucose then diminishes the need for protein to be used as a fuel source, preserving your all-important muscle mass.

Table 4.1 summarizes the amount of fuel provided by the various sources of carbohydrates, protein, and fat stored in your body.

Essentially, fat and glycogen are the major fuels that the body uses for energy

4.1

CALORIES PROVIDED BY BODY FUEL STORES

BODY FUEL STORES	CALORIES
Carbohydrate Stores	
Blood glucose	80
Liver glycogen	400
Muscle glycogen	1,400–1,800
Fat Stores	
Blood fatty acids	7
Serum triglycerides	75
Muscle triglycerides	2,700
Adipose tissue triglycerides	80,000
Protein Stores	
Muscle protein	30,000

during training. Exercise intensity, which can be measured as a percentage of your heart rate as a percentage of your VO_2 max, is particularly important in determining which of these two fuels your body prefers. Generally, the harder you train, the more carbohydrates you burn. Interval training in which you take your heart rate to higher intensities burns a significant amount of carbohydrates. When you go out for a nice steady swim or ride at an intensity you can maintain for several hours, fat provides a nice amount of fuel. Training simply activates the energy system that can best meet the fuel demands of your training session. It is your job to ensure that this energy system is well supplied. During most types of endurance training sessions, you will burn a mix of both carbohydrates and fat. During high intensity exercise you burn a greater percentage of carbohydrates, and during lower intensity exercise you burn a greater percentage of fat.

THE THREE ENERGY SYSTEMS

The three energy systems in your body are activated by the type and amount of fuel that can best meet the energy demands of your training session. If your body needs carbohydrates quickly, then the lactic acid system is activated. If your body requires a steady supply of fat, the aerobic lipolytic system is activated. The ATP-CP system can be activated for an all-out sprint effort at the end of a race. Table 4.2 summarizes the characteristics of these energy systems.

Let's take a look at how training activates the two anaerobic fuel systems. The ATP-CP system, which is the first of two anaerobic energy systems, provides a short-lived and limited fuel supply. During shorter, high intensity sprint events there is a rapid activation of both the ATP-CP and the anaerobic glycolysis systems. ATP and CP provide up to ten seconds of energy. Then the anaerobic glycolysis or lactic acid system supplies glucose, mainly from muscle glycogen, to be used for fuel. Muscle glycogen is broken down rapidly when exercise is intense, and eventually the demand for ATP exceeds the body's readily available supply. Performance is also limited by the excess production of lactic acid that is a byproduct of activating this energy system. There is a gradual increase in muscle acidity, which causes a decrease in the force of muscle contraction. If you have ever sprinted at the end of a race or completed a sprint finish at the end of a bike ride, you have activated this energy system.

These anaerobic energy systems are also utilized when high intensity exercise bouts are part of aerobic events, such as high intensity or all-out efforts during a bike race, marathon, or ski event. Intermittent exercise as seen during interval training uses an extended combination of aerobic and anaerobic exercise—also resulting in a rapid breakdown of muscle glycogen. High intensity, repeated resistance training also depletes your muscle glycogen stores.

4.2

CHARACTERISTICS OF THE BODY'S ENERGY SYSTEMS

ANAEROBIC SYSTEMS

ATP-CP System	**Anaerobic Glycolysis (Lactic Acid System)**
Highest rate of ATP production	High rate ATP production
Very limited supply of ATP lasting 6–10 seconds	Limited supply ATP lasting 2 minutes
Highest power output and intensity level	High power output and intensity level
Uses ATP and creatine phosphate stored in body	Uses ATP, creatine phosphate, and muscle glycogen for fuel
Develops explosive power	Develops lactate tolerance

AEROBIC SYSTEMS

Glycolytic	**Glycolytic and Lipolytic**
15–90 minutes exercise	*More than 90 minutes exercise*
Low rate of ATP production	Lowest rate of ATP production
High supply ATP	High supply ATP
Low power production	Lowest power output
Lower intensity	Lowest intensity level
15–30 minutes exercise: uses muscle glycogen and blood glucose for energy	Longer than 90 minutes exercise: uses muscle glycogen, blood glucose, intramuscular fat, and adipose tissue fat for energy
60–90 minutes exercise: uses muscle glycogen, blood glucose, and intramuscular fat for energy	

When you train with a heart rate monitor, it provides the feedback you require to perform the appropriate training session for that day in order to stay within a specific heart rate zone. This heart rate monitor can also provide you with feedback on the mix of fuels you would burn during exercise. Logically, aerobic exercise such as a nice steady bike ride, run, or swim does not seem to cause fuel depletion as quickly as high intensity exercise and therefore can be sustained longer.

The aerobic system is the third energy system and is designed to supply fuel for longer periods of time. The reason you can exercise longer is because exercise at low to moderate intensity of less than 60 percent maximum heart rate is fueled mainly by your fat stores. As you become more highly trained, changes in your hormone levels cause your fat tissue to release fatty acids in the bloodstream. These fatty acids, and fat stored in your muscles, then fuel your low intensity efforts and are a seemingly endless supply of energy. However, glycogen is still a fuel supply during these lower intensity efforts and eventually carbohydrate stores will run too low for training to continue.

The aerobic system also supplies fuel during moderate intensity exercise at about 60 to 80 percent of your maximum heart rate, and muscle glycogen and blood glucose stores supply about half of your energy needs. The other half of your energy needs come mainly from fat, and a very small amount comes from protein. Exercise maintained at this level is also limited by your carbohydrate stores. Even at the lower end of moderate intensity exercise, you will eventually run low on glycogen. Depletion may not occur quickly, but it will happen.

Eventually, your aerobic system cannot fully meet the demands of your training as exercise intensity increases. When you train at even higher intensities such as levels exceeding 80 percent of your maximum heart rate, fat cannot be utilized effectively as a fuel and provides less than 25 percent of your energy needs. This is because your fat stores cannot be broken down quickly enough to produce ATP at the faster rate required. To meet these energy demands, fuel is provided mainly by your carbohydrate stores so that ATP can be quickly supplied. As would be expected, your production of lactic acid increases at this higher intensity. Lactic acid also impedes the release of fat as an energy source. When you exercise at 90 to 95 percent of your maximum heart rate, your body relies essentially on glucose for energy.

To keep things simple, you can also view how your body utilizes fat and carbohydrates from the perspective of how long you train. The longer you train, the more fat supplies fuel for your efforts. Fat can only be used effectively as the major fuel source at up to 60 to 70 percent of your VO_2 max. Even at lower exercise intensities, a certain level of carbohydrates are also needed for fat to be burned as energy. Therefore, when you train during longer sessions, your exercise intensity must decrease as muscle glycogen stores run low. For longer duration exercise of four to six hours, which requires lower intensities in order to be sustained, as much as 60 to 70 percent of all the fuel burned can come from fat.

But it is important for you to appreciate, as an endurance athlete, that despite the variation in fuel burned at different levels of exercise intensity, muscle glycogen remains a significant fuel for most types of endurance training. As previously mentioned, even in longer events where the slower pace accommodates fat burning, muscle glycogen stores can eventually become depleted.

What fuel your body will burn is also determined by your fitness level. Training has many benefits in terms of fuel usage. When you are fit, your body becomes more efficient at producing energy aerobically at a given intensity. This allows you to maintain this intensity at a lower percentage of your maximum heart rate. Consequently, you burn more fat and less glycogen, saving your much more limited glycogen stores. This adaptation partly explains how elite athletes can tolerate intense exercise levels without hitting the wall.

Adaptations to training can also occur with changes in lactic acid accumulation. For example, untrained individuals could begin to accumulate blood lactic acid at 50 to 60 percent of their maximal aerobic capacity. Training can bump this lactate threshold up to 70 to 75 percent, or even higher in elite athletes. Because lactic acid interferes with fat burning and speeds up muscle glycogen use, having a higher lactate

Your VO$_2$ Max and Lactate Threshold

Without oxygen, training is not possible. The harder you exercise, the more oxygen your body requires to function. Eventually you will reach a level beyond which you cannot increase your oxygen use. This point where your oxygen consumption plateaus is called maximal oxygen consumption or VO$_2$ max. An athlete with a high VO$_2$ max is considered to have a greater endurance capacity than an athlete with a lower VO$_2$ max.

VO$_2$ max is as scientific as it sounds. It is actually a measurement of your aerobic capacity, or the amount of oxygen your muscles can extract from the bloodstream. Unfortunately, your ultimate aerobic capacity or VO$_2$ max is mainly determined by genetics. But you can follow a training program that will enable you to reach your full oxygen capacity potential and subsequently perform your best.

Highly trained athletes can maintain maximal aerobic capacity for only several minutes. Most of the time, you are exercising at a percentage of your maximal aerobic capacity, often called percentage of VO$_2$ max. Because many athletes have not undergone the scientific testing available to determine VO$_2$ max, exercise intensity is often expressed as a percentage of maximal heart rate. Many athletes are familiar with their maximal heart rate as they train with a heart rate monitor.

Lactate threshold is another scientific measurement that refers to a specific percentage of VO$_2$ max. Like VO$_2$ max, the level at which lactate threshold occurs varies among athletes. During exercise of increasing intensity, a byproduct called lactic acid is produced. The point at which excess lactic acid begins to accumulate in your blood is referred to as the lactate threshold. The lactate threshold is usually expressed as a percentage of VO_2 max, but can also be expressed as a percentage of maximal heart rate. Every athlete has his or her own lactate threshold—your lactate threshold may be at 80 percent of your maximal heart rate.

Lactate threshold is also an important indicator of athletic performance. Basically it measures an athlete's ability to sustain a high rate of energy expenditure without being limited by fatigue. An athlete with a lactate threshold at 75 percent of VO_2 max should have better endurance potential than an athlete with the same VO_2 max and lactate threshold at 70 percent. This is because the higher lactate threshold allows the athlete to work closer to his aerobic capacity. In fact, lactate threshold is often a better predictor of endurance performance ability than VO_2 max.

Genetics influences your lactate threshold, but so does training. Good training programs are designed to increase your lactate tolerance. Both your VO_2 max and lactate threshold can be measured from a graded exercise test on a bicycle or treadmill. Follow-up testing can determine how these performance measurements have responded to your current training program. ■

threshold allows you to use more fat and less glycogen at the same exercise intensity. Well-designed programs that increase your lactic acid tolerance play an important role in helping you achieve your competition goals.

Endurance training has one other added benefit. It increases your muscle storage capacity of glycogen. Your muscle glycogen is not only used at a slower rate when you are trained, but you also begin exercise with higher glycogen stores. All these adaptations result in more stored fuel, more efficient use of fuel, and a higher fatigue threshold.

Your training program will determine the intensity and duration of your training sessions. What is most important is that you match your nutrition choices with your training efforts so that you can recover on a daily basis. One masters cyclist felt that he had to go for long rides at a low intensity and not consume carbohydrates in order to lose unwanted body fat. Avoiding carbohydrates during prolonged exercise is not necessary for becoming a lean athlete. You are always burning a combination of carbohydrates and fat. Ultimately what supports your weight loss efforts is the calories you burn simply from training. This assists you in creating a mild calorie deficit that eventually results in a healthy rate of body fat loss. This cyclist also placed undue stress upon his body by not consuming enough carbohydrates during exercise when his muscle glycogen stores did eventually run low. Many athletes who practice this unadvised technique experience low energy levels and extreme hunger later in the day.

ENERGY FOR ENDURANCE TRAINING

While this chapter will outline your absolute carbohydrate, protein, and fat requirements for endurance training, it is also important to appreciate how your daily training affects your energy requirements. Estimating energy needs is not a precise science, but there are some general indicators that can give you an appreciation of just how high your calorie needs may be for daily recovery from one training session to the next. Energy needs are presented as the amount of calories required per pound of weight. Your energy requirements can vary daily as your training program dictates. With endurance training, it is best not to fall short on your calorie intake. Several days in a row of not recharging your batteries may result in some unplanned rest and days off, which can hamper your competition goals.

Mild activity with no purposeful exercise or training: 12–14 calories per pound.
Moderate activity with up to one hour daily of moderate intensity exercise: 15–17 calories per pound.

High activity of one to two hours daily of moderate intensity: 18–24 calories
  per pound.

Very high activity of several hours training daily: 25–30 calories per pound.

Carbohydrates: The Recovery Fuel

While you may have "hit the wall" during a training session and experienced the symptoms of glycogen depletion during a single training session, the symptoms of gradual
glycogen depletion related to successive days of heavy training can be much more subtle. These symptoms can creep up over a week's time or longer, producing feelings of
sluggishness or heaviness. Besides general lethargy, you may put out an increased effort
during training and find it difficult to maintain a given intensity. Your morning swim
that is normally a breeze may make you feel like you are swimming through quicksand.

Numerous scientific studies have measured that a diet adequate in carbohydrates
is superior in building, maintaining, and replenishing muscle glycogen stores. The
amount of carbohydrates you consume in your diet directly affects the amount of
glycogen you store in your muscles and liver. Inadequate intake of carbohydrates will
lead to only partial replenishment of muscle glycogen stores. If this incomplete
replenishment occurs from one day to the next, glycogen stores are gradually depleted
over a week or more, and your training will suffer. Adequate recovery allows you to
start the next training session, whether it is three, six, twelve, or twenty-four hours
away, with optimal fuel to complete the exercise at the desired duration and intensity spelled out in your training program.

Carbohydrate Requirements: Grams Matter!

Carbohydrate recommendations are often expressed as a percentage of total calories.
This is appropriate for general recommendations for the community, when the goal is
to decrease unwanted fat intake and to increase carbohydrates from whole grains,
fruits and vegetables. However, for endurance athletes, it is more appropriate to express
carbohydrate needs as grams per pound of weight based on the intensity and duration

of the training session. Your muscles require an absolute amount of carbohydrate to recover sufficiently, particularly after long and intense training sessions such as a three-hour bike ride or two hours of interval swimming early in the morning.

The ceiling for daily carbohydrate consumption, at which point your muscle storage capacity has been reached, is 4.5–5.5 grams of carbohydrates for every pound of weight. Depending on the size of the athlete, this translates to about 500–700 grams of carbohydrates daily. Most endurance athletes who meet both their energy and carbohydrate needs will average about 60 percent carbohydrate calories in their training diets. But depending on whether an athlete is interested in restricting calories or has very high energy needs, he could consume anywhere from 50 to 70 percent of calories from carbohydrates, while still consuming an adequate total amount of carbohydrate grams. Typically, as an endurance athlete you will have to consume greater quantities of carbohydrates than most people, including athletes participating in sports that do not have these high fuel demands.

Your absolute carbohydrate intake can be fine-tuned and adjusted daily according to your current training load and ability to recover. With successive days of heavy training you would clearly benefit from the high end of the recommended amounts. Moderate training sessions may not require quite as many carbohydrates. Also keep in mind that rest days are still your "catch-up" recovery days during which you should consume enough carbohydrates to allow for adequate replenishment, without the concern of burning additional carbohydrate stores with exercise. Table 4.3 outlines the daily carbohydrate requirements for training sessions of varying intensity and duration. When planning your daily carbohydrate intake, you should consider not only that day's training, but also your goals for the next day and how well you have recovered from the previous day's session.

Practical Carbohydrate Issues

As an endurance athlete you must make a concerted effort to obtain adequate amounts of carbohydrates at specific times in portions that may exceed your appetite

4.3

DAILY CARBOHYDRATE REQUIREMENTS

Training Regimen	Carbohydrate Requirements (per pound of weight)
Extremely prolonged: Greater than 3–6 hours daily Moderate/high intensity	4.5–5.5 g/lb.
Prolonged: Greater than 90 minutes daily Moderate/high intensity	3.0–4.5 g/lb.
Moderate duration: Moderate intensity under 1 hour Low intensity for several hours	2.25–3.0 g/lb.
Sedentary adult	0.4 g/lb.

and hunger levels, and exceed the amounts of certain nutrients that are typically provided in the North American diet. While wholesome carbohydrates are appreciated for their nutritional content, you often will need to focus on carbohydrate-rich foods that are appealing, convenient, and carbohydrate dense for a given serving.

Food tables that provide carbohydrate portions for 30-gram servings are provided in Chapter 6, which covers meal planning and provides practical guidelines for putting together a top sports diet. You can match up these carbohydrate amounts to provide you with the total grams of carbohydrates required for training on a given day. A 160-pound triathlete may require up to 480 grams of carbohydrates on an easy one-hour recovery day, but need a full 720 grams of carbohydrates on a training day that includes a five-hour bike ride. Consuming 500 grams of carbohydrates is simpler than consuming 700 grams, as attaining the higher carbohydrate amount would likely require more structure and planning. This food system outlined in Chapter 6 provides you with the flexibility to emphasize various carbohydrate sources from one day to the next depending on your food preferences, cravings, and schedule. However, for those very high carbohydrate days, you may want to consider the following suggestions:

- Sports bars or energy bars are a concentrated and convenient source of carbohydrates, supplying up to 50 grams per serving. They travel well and can be consumed quickly between training sessions or on the way back to work. But do keep in mind that these bars are often vitamin and mineral fortified. Make sure that you do not consume too high of doses of these nutrients simply by over-consuming sports bars.

- Low fiber carbohydrate foods may be more practical when carbohydrates need to be consumed in very large amounts. They can be consumed in combination with higher fiber items. Choices include large bagels, calorie-dense cereals, fruit juices, jams, honey, and syrup.

- A well-timed yogurt with fruit, low fat milkshake, or fruit smoothie can up your carbohydrate intake considerably and provide needed fluid as well. They also taste good!

- High carbohydrate supplement drinks or meal replacements may also be a convenient source of carbohydrates. They are easy to carry and quickly consumed.

- Desserts can be part of a nutritious diet. Some carbohydrate dense choices include sherbet, sorbet, and frozen yogurt topped with fruit.

- Meeting your daily carbohydrate intake often requires consuming between-meal snacks and "grazing" throughout the day. Carbohydrate rich foods should comprise at least half of your meals and snacks. Low fiber choices may work best when food is consumed close to the start of exercise.

- Keep an eye out for carbohydrate foods that are also high in fat (often unhealthy fats) such as croissants, creamed or deep fried vegetables, doughnuts, French toast, fried rice, muffins, pancakes, pastries, potato chips, snack crackers, and popcorn popped with oil.

Obtaining the total grams of carbohydrates that you require to match your training may be your biggest nutritional challenge of the day. While you want to emphasize fruits, vegetables, and whole grains, higher carbohydrate needs for more intense and longer training may require that you incorporate less filling but carbohydrate dense foods into your diet. Meeting these carbohydrate amounts requires planning and a good appetite.

Protein and Your Recovery Requirements

While carbohydrate intake is clearly emphasized in an endurance sports diet, your training program also increases your need for protein. You may find it ironic that your protein requirements often exceed those of strength and power athletes. But you may also find it comforting to realize that your elevated protein requirements are easily met by choosing a well-balanced sports diet. Protein powder and special supplements really are not necessary for your training program. Table 4.4 outlines the protein requirements of endurance athletes.

Because endurance training depletes carbohydrate reserves, protein may become a viable fuel source during longer training sessions. When glycogen runs low, amino acids stored in the muscle can be converted to glucose, possibly supplying up to 15 percent of your fuel usage. This is a significant increase as protein supplies only 5 percent of your energy needs when glycogen stores are adequate. Not consuming enough carbohydrates and calories will limit your glycogen stores prior to exercise and increase your use of protein during exercise. Relatively minor protein losses have

4.4

DAILY PROTEIN REQUIREMENTS

Exercise Type	Protein Requirements (per lb. of weight)
Endurance athlete:	
Moderate training	0.45 g/lb.
Heavy training	0.50–0.75 g/lb.
Very intense training	0.8–0.9 g/lb.
Growing teenage athlete	0.8–0.9 g/lb.
Athlete restricting calories	0.8–0.9 g/lb.
Strength training phase of training:	
Experienced	0.5–0.7 g/lb.
Novice	0.8 g/lb.
Maximum recommended amount for extreme exercise loads	1.0 g/lb.

been found in the urine after exercise and in sweat. Therefore, protein in your diet is required to replace protein burned for fuel during longer and depleting training sessions and to repair exercise-induced muscle damage.

If strength training is a component of your program, your protein requirements are not significantly elevated above your endurance training requirements during this phase. Though traditionally strength training athletes have consumed large amounts of protein in hopes of building more muscle mass, actual protein requirements for building this tissue are relatively small.

What is most important for you to appreciate is that your elevated protein requirements are easily met by a well-planned sports diet. For endurance athletes consuming enough calories to meet their energy needs, this often translates into an increased protein intake. The typical North American diet supplies about 12 to 20 percent of calories from protein. When calories go up, the percentage from protein often remains constant, and the total grams of protein you consume increases. Adequate protein intake may only be a concern for a poorly planned vegetarian diet or athletes following a calorie restriction.

Average protein intakes for most endurance athletes range from 70 to 200 grams daily depending on their caloric intake. Consider how easy it is to meet your daily protein requirements. Having some peanut butter and cereal with milk for breakfast, a turkey sandwich for lunch, and a stir-fry of lean red meat and rice for dinner will supply about 90 grams of protein. You will obtain additional protein from between-meal snacks. Foods such as whole grains and vegetables, which are not as concentrated in protein, still contribute to your total protein intake and can provide moderate amounts over the course of a day that supplement your intake of more concentrated protein foods.

Protein Supplements

Marketing of whole protein and amino acid supplements is heavily targeted toward endurance athletes as well as strength athletes. Supporters of amino acid supplementation claim that these products are more readily digested and absorbed than the protein found in foods. This simply is false, as your body is well equipped to handle protein from whole foods by secreting a number of enzymes that renders amino acid absorption at 90 percent effectiveness. Amino acid supplements are also marketed as repairing damaged muscle more quickly. Again, there is no evidence to support this claim. While what you consume in the few hours after exercise can facilitate muscle recovery, full post-exercise muscle repair cannot be completed in minutes, further invalidating the claims made about these products.

There are a variety of claims surrounding amino acid supplementation. For example, many products marketed to body builders claim to build muscle and burn fat. Arginine and ornithine are two such promoted amino acids. Supposedly they stimulate the secretion of growth hormone, which then increases muscle mass. In fact, what seems to occur is that large amounts of these amino acids are needed to promote a temporary rise in growth hormone. In addition, there is no proof that this rise results in increased muscle mass. There is currently no sound scientific data to support that supplementing with these amino acids produces this muscle-building effect.

Endurance athletes may also be sold on three amino acids—leucine, isoleucine, and valine, often referred to as branched chain amino acids due to their structure. When protein is required for energy during endurance exercise, branched chain amino acids are converted to glucose. You can minimize the use of branched chain amino acids as a fuel source by beginning exercise with adequate carbohydrate stores. Regardless, obtaining branched chain amino acids from foods before and after endurance exercise is fairly simple. Some foods high in branched chain amino acids include many liquid protein-carbohydrate recovery supplements, milk and yogurt, fish, poultry, and lean red meat.

It is also important for you to appreciate that amino acid or protein metabolism is very complex. It is affected by a variety of factors including amino acid concentration in the blood, competition with other available amino acids, and the presence of other nutrients. Amino acid mixtures could potentially lead to nutritional imbalances, as an excess of one amino acid may negatively affect the absorption of another. Amino acid supplement dosing may also be misleading. A bottle listing up to 500 milligrams in a capsule actually contains only 0.5 grams, or less than one gram, of amino acids, whereas only one ounce of chicken contains 7,000 milligrams, or 7 grams of amino acids in the form of whole protein. Clearly, amino acid supplements cannot meet the dosing found in a compact source of natural protein.

Dangers of Excess Protein

A well-balanced diet with adequate calories and up to 15 percent protein provides enough grams of protein for the muscle growth and repair required after endurance training. Protein that is consumed in excess of your requirements is simply excess calories and is then burned for energy or stored as fat. Converting protein to fuel for exercise is inefficient when compared to carbohydrates, which are much more easily burned for energy. There are other negative effects from consuming excess protein. Protein from both food and supplements increases your need for fluid, as your kidneys require more water to eliminate the end products of protein metabolism. Individuals with liver or kidney problems are also susceptible to negative effects of excessive dietary protein. Excess dietary protein leads to urinary excretion of calcium and can possibly contribute to the development of osteoporosis. While food sources of protein are best, they can also contribute substantial amounts of fat and cholesterol to the diet. Consuming excess protein can mean taking in excess fat and cholesterol and increasing your risk of heart disease and other health problems. You should be selective regarding the type of protein foods you eat. There are plenty of low fat, animal protein food sources to choose from and plenty of healthy plant proteins as well.

Your protein needs for endurance training, muscle repair, and other important protein functions are easily met through a well-planned diet adequate in calories. The key is to obtain adequate amounts of quality protein sources throughout the day and to consume enough calories so that protein is not burned for energy.

Fat Intake and Fuel Requirements

Because endurance athletes burn a large percentage of fat as fuel during endurance exercise, you may wonder if increasing your fat intake will improve your performance. When you are highly trained and well fed, muscle glycogen may provide up to 1,800 calories of fuel. In contrast, adipose tissue is the largest energy reserve in your body, ranging from 50,000 to more than 100,000 stored calories in some athletes. In order to utilize fat effectively as a fuel source, fatty acids must leave these fat stores and be transported in the blood to your exercising muscles. But while many athletes may be very focused on their level of adipose tissue fat, there is another very important source of stored body fat. Intramuscular triglycerides (IMTG) can provide as much as 2,700–3,100 calories of stored energy. Your endurance training program increases your stores of IMTG, as can eating adequate fat in your diet.

In a recent study, researchers examined the effects of three diets providing varying amounts of fat. Seven endurance cyclists were tested. Their regular diet of about 32 percent fat and 58 percent carbohydrates was the control diet. The two test diets were a 22% fat and 68% carbohydrate diet, and an extremely low fat diet of 2% fat and 88% carbohydrates. All three diets provided between 4,200 and 4,400 calories, 10% of which came from protein. Subjects followed each diet for seven days and exercised two hours daily on days two through six of the diet protocol.

With the extreme 2% fat diet, researchers found a reduction in body fat oxidation, which they felt reflected decreased IMTG oxidation. Their data also suggest that the very low fat diet also reduced stores of IMTG and increased muscle glycogen levels. However, increasing the diet from 22% fat to 32% fat did not significantly increase IMTG, though muscle glycogen levels were higher on the 22% fat diet as it provided more carbohydrates. What is clear from this data is that extremely low fat diets are not appropriate for optimal IMTG stores. Just what level of fat is needed is not absolutely certain and will be determined from future research.

We do know for certain that endurance training stimulates the body to burn more fat during exercise. There is an increase in the level of fat-burning enzymes, and

increasing your lactate threshold also improves your ability to utilize fat, thus sparing the more limited muscle glycogen. As exercise increases to about 65 percent of
VO_2 max, more of the fat burned for fuel is supplied by muscle triglycerides. So just
as you need to replace glycogen stores by consuming sufficient dietary carbohydrates, an adequate fat intake will also replenish these muscle triglyceride stores.

The bottom line advice is simple—don't follow an overly restrictive low fat diet.
Because of your increased energy needs, obtaining 20 to 25 percent of your daily
caloric intake from fat will provide more than enough total grams of fat (remember
percentages are all relative). Dietary fat is also a concentrated source of energy. Once
your carbohydrate requirements have been met, you may find that beefing up your
diet with healthy fats (see Chapter 2) will simply give you the calories you need to
meet your high energy requirements. Adding healthy oils to foods and munching on
nuts and seeds will not add much volume to your diet, but often provides needed
calories and essential fatty acids.

While your recovery does depend upon the right balance of carbohydrates, protein,
and fat for your training that day, there are several strategies that can fine-tune and
highly accentuate the recovery process. Just as a large part of your daily sports diet
hinges on your carbohydrate intake, the early recovery process after exercise hinges
on this important nutrient, among others, as well.

Daily Recovery

Overall, your daily recovery hinges on obtaining enough calories in your diet to
replace the fuels you burned and to support your daily life activities. Because of the
relatively limited supply of glycogen in the body, and the integral role of glycogen
in supplying fuel during all types of endurance training, carbohydrates are important nutrients for the endurance athlete. Carbohydrates are needed to synthesize
glycogen, and you must consume enough total grams of carbohydrates to fully
replenish stores. It is also important that the amount of carbohydrates you consume
matches your training for that day.

Protein is needed for recovery to build and repair muscle tissue. Adequate protein in your diet will also maintain a strong immune system. After arduous training sessions, you may also need to replace protein burned for fuel. Your elevated protein requirements are easily met through a well-planned diet that is adequate in calories.

Dietary fat is also part of your recovery plan. About 20 to 25 percent of your calories should come from fat to provide essential fatty acids, energy, and to replace intramuscular triglyceride stores. Fat intake can also be increased once carbohydrate and protein intake is adequate to provide calories for endurance athletes with very high energy needs.

Fine-tuning the Recovery Process

Carbohydrate, Protein, Fluid, and Sodium Immediately after Exercise

While the most important factor affecting daily muscle glycogen recovery is the total amount of carbohydrates consumed, eating carbohydrates in the two hours after training can speed up the recovery process and provide you with a good jump start toward total carbohydrate replenishment. Several scientific studies have resulted in the development of the recommendation to consume anywhere from 0.5 to 0.7 grams of carbohydrates per pound of body weight within thirty minutes of completing endurance exercise. One study demonstrated that subjects fed carbohydrates a full two hours after exercise synthesized the carbohydrates into glycogen 45 percent more slowly than subjects fed carbohydrates immediately after exercise. It appears that muscle glycogen storage is slightly enhanced two hours after exercise, during which time the muscle has a greater capacity to take up blood glucose and is more sensitive to insulin, the hormone that brings glucose into the cells.

Studies have shown that both liquid and solid carbohydrates are adequate in refueling the body after endurance exercise. However, emphasizing higher glycemic carbohydrate foods that elicit a higher insulin response, such as sports nutrition supplements, breads, and cereals, may enhance glycogen resynthesis. A list of high glycemic foods is provided in Appendix A.

For the rest of the day, carbohydrates can be consumed as a series of snacks or a few larger meals depending on your training schedule and preferences. Both eating styles will sufficiently promote glycogen recovery if the total amount of carbohydrates consumed is adequate. Eating a balanced mix of low glycemic and high glycemic carbohydrates throughout the day will support the glycogen recovery process. But consuming an adequate amount of total carbohydrate grams over the 24-hour period is still your most important carbohydrate recovery strategy.

There has been a fair amount of debate regarding the benefits of adding protein to the recovery carbohydrate snack immediately after exercise. Study results have varied depending on whether or not the protein provided additional calories or whether researchers provided the same amount of calories when comparing a carbohydrate-only dose to a carbohydrate and protein combination dose. What is certain is that having protein comprise about one-fourth of your recovery snack will not compromise your muscle glycogen recovery. Consuming some protein immediately after exercise may also speed up the repair of muscle tissue and provide important nutrients for your immune system. It will also send you on your way to optimizing your protein intake until the next training session.

Of course, rehydration is also a top priority after endurance training as athletes typically replace only three-fourths of their sweat losses during training. Your goal is to fully restore fluid losses from one training session to the next while keeping in mind that thirst is not a reliable indicator of fluid losses. You are already dehydrated when you are thirsty, and the thirst mechanism will shut down before you have sufficiently replaced all your fluid losses. Try to consume up to three cups of fluid for every pound of weight lost after training. Sixteen ounces actually replaces a fluid loss of two pounds, but the higher volume of 24 ounces will replace both sweat and subsequent urine losses.

Pay attention to what stimulates your desire to drink. You may prefer a sweeter product or perhaps something a bit salty. The temperature of the drink may also affect the volume of fluid you consume. It makes sense that a cool drink would be more palatable, particularly in hot weather, while it may be difficult to drink large amounts of a very cold beverage.

Some athletes may feel reluctant to weigh themselves before and after every training session. You may also not have a scale available every time you train. What you can do is obtain pre- and post-exercise weights after specific types of training sessions. For example, you may determine that you replace only 50 percent of your fluid needs during high intensity training, whereas you meet 80 percent of your fluid requirements during lower intensity exercise when it may be easier to reach for and consume fluid. Once you have established the replenishment levels of your best drinking efforts, you can then develop a system for rehydrating after exercise. You may also want to determine what your typical fluid losses are for specific types of environmental conditions. Of course, you can also check the color of your urine to evaluate your hydration efforts. Clear urine can reflect adequate hydration. But on days when you know you are to train or compete in more extreme conditions, you may want to carefully check your weight before and after exercise.

Sodium or salt may not only stimulate your drive to drink but can also enhance the rehydration process. Generally, sweating results in large fluid losses and relatively small sodium losses. When you finish exercise, your blood volume and total body water is reduced, while there is a mild increase in blood concentration and its sodium content. When you consume large amounts of plain water after exercise, you dilute your blood before your full blood volume has been restored. This diluting effect will shut down the thirst mechanism, and you will urinate to bring the concentration of the blood to a normal level. The end result is that you have produced a large amount of dilute urine before you are fully rehydrated.

You can offset this negative effect by consuming some sodium or salt after exercise. A series of studies determined that rehydrating with drinks higher in sodium produced significantly lower urine losses than low sodium drinks, indicating that more of the fluid consumed was retained for hydration. Therefore, it is recommended that when your fluid losses are significant, that you replace sodium losses

What about Fat Loading?

Several well-designed published fat studies performed at the Australian Institute of Sport in Canberra have shed some more light on fat metabolism during exercise. These studies were designed to test the hypothesis that athletes may be able to adapt to a high fat diet for three to five days prior to an event, then carbohydrate load in the forty-eight hours before competition. A short-term diet is preferred, as longer-term high fat diets are difficult to follow, would not allow for optimal training, and may have adverse health effects. Hopefully, this technique would both maximize glycogen stores before competition and optimize the muscle's capacity for fat oxidation during endurance exercise. These studies concluded with a time trial performance test to better mimic real athletic conditions.

In the first such study, researchers compared a high carbohydrate diet (4.46 g/lb. wt.) to high fat diet (1.8 g fat/lb. and 1.1 g CHO/lb.) consumed for five days. Both diets were equal in calories, and the eight subjects who were competitive cyclists or triathletes completed supervised training while on the diets. Day six consisted of rest and ingestion of a high carbohydrate diet. On day seven the well-trained subjects cycled at 70 percent VO_2 max for two hours and completed a time trial lasting approximately thirty minutes. In this initial study, the exercise test was conducted after an overnight fast, and the subjects consumed only water during the exercise.

Researchers found that on the high fat diet there was a drastic reduction in muscle glycogen concentration. But one day on the high carbohydrate diet (day six) restored muscle glycogen levels, though levels were still below those on the high carbohydrate diet. During the two-hour cycling test, less muscle glycogen was used for fuel on the fat adaptation diet—indicating glycogen sparing. It was not measured if the increased fat burned during exercise was from IMTG. However, despite these fat adaptations, there was not a statistically significant difference in the time trial performance between the two diets, though there was a trend toward improved performance on the high fat diet.

In the second study, the design was similar. Subject consumed either the high fat or high carbohydrate diet for five days. This was followed by one day of a high carbohydrate diet and rest. The only difference was that subjects consumed a high carbohydrate pre-exercise meal two hours prior to the two-hour cycling bout and time trial and consumed a specified amount of a carbohydrate-electrolyte beverage every twenty minutes during exercise.

It was expected that this carbohydrate intake would suppress fat utilization during exercise.

Compared to the first study, the overall rate of fat utilization was lower. But there was still an increase in total fat oxidation following the fat adaptation diet when compared to the high carbohydrate diet. Researchers felt that there were persistent adaptations to the short-term high fat diet, even when carbohydrates were consumed before and during exercise. However, the time trial did not find any performance advantage with the high fat diet.

In a third fat adaptation study, researchers looked at ultraendurance exercise, as fat metabolism has a greater impact on this type of exercise. Seven trained cyclists consumed the same high fat diet or an even higher carbohydrate diet (5 g/lb. wt.) for six days. A day of rest and consumption of a high carbohydrate diet followed this

(continued on page 84)

(continued from page 83)
diet. The next day subjects consumed a high carbohydrate pre-exercise meal and cycled for four hours at 65 percent VO_2 max followed by a one-hour time trial. The high fat diet did result in greater fat utilization during exercise. There was an increase in mean power output during the time trial after the fat adaptation diet, but there was no statistical difference between the two groups in the distance covered during the one-hour cycling time trial, though there was a 4 percent improvement with the high fat diet.

So Should You Fat Load?

Based on this data, advising endurance athletes to fat load would be very preliminary advice. What is likely is that there are some individuals who do respond better to fat loading than others. On the other hand, study data indicate that some individuals could have impairment of exercise capacity with a fat loading diet, especially when training at higher heart rates. Often race situations necessitate higher intensity effects due to race strategy, the breakaway tactics of your competitors, varying terrain, and intense efforts to the finish. And while there was glycogen sparing on the fat loading diet, consuming carbohydrates during exercise seemed to offset any benefit derived, up to about 2.5 hours of exercise. More research should help clarify what athletic events could benefit from a safe and effective fat-loading dietary protocol. It is also necessary that the desired pre-race training can be maintained while on the higher fat diet. What really remains to be determined with future research is if some individuals benefit from fat loading before ultra-endurance exercise, and to determine the characteristics of responders and non-responders. ■

as well. It also appears that some individuals may have greater sodium sweat losses than others, so consuming sodium after exercise may be prudent unless medically contraindicated. Some athletes may actually require up to several grams of sodium over the course of the day after endurance training in hot weather. Guidelines for promoting immediate post-exercise nutritional recovery are:

- Consume at least 0.5 grams carbohydrates per pound of weight; consider adding 10–15 grams of protein if desired. Drink 24 ounces of fluid for every pound of weight lost during exercise. If fluid losses are significant, consume moderate amounts of sodium after exercise. Start with several hundred milligrams of sodium and incorporate sodium into your diet throughout the day.
- Experiment to find your favorite recovery snack/drink combination(s) from foods and sports supplements. You may enjoy a powdered milk- or soy-based shake that can be mixed with juice or prefer a large glass of juice with cereal and milk, while on other days a bagel with jam combined with a recovery drink can work for you as well.
- Sports drinks are formulated for tolerable consumption during exercise, not post exercise. A 150-pound athlete requires 75 grams of carbohydrates, which translates to 40 ounces of a sports drink. Sports drinks are also relatively low in sodium. You may consider adding one-fourth to one-half teaspoon of salt to your total fluid intake. However, this may not be your most effective recovery fluid choice.
- Recovery products that are concentrated in carbohydrates, providing anywhere from 50 to 100 grams per 16-ounce serving, are also available. Some of these products also provide up to 25 grams of protein per serving. Sports tubes that provide only protein are also available and can be consumed with a high carbohydrate source.
- Other sports nutrition products such as gels and bars can be consumed conveniently after exercise. They should be taken with plenty of fluid, including those that provide carbohydrates.

- Experiment with your own low fat shake and smoothie recipes made from dairy milk, yogurt, soy milk, or juice, and fresh or frozen fruit for a hydrating carbohydrate and protein combination.
- Fruit flavored yogurt can make a great recovery snack with juice or a granola bar.
- Cereal with milk and fruit provides a good protein and carbohydrate combination.
- Monitor your body weight pre- and post-exercise to determine how well you replace fluid during exercise and what volume you need to consume to replace fluid losses.
- Make sure you have fluids that you like and that are at your preferred temperature readily available after exercise.
- Have some salty foods, or add salt to your meals and snacks after exercise to replace sodium losses, especially when you have lost more than 2 quarts of fluid overall during exercise.
- Be organized and plan your recovery drinks and snacks after intense or long training sessions.
- Limit caffeine-containing beverages after exercise to optimize fluid replacement. Consume alcohol only after fluid balance has been restored, if at all.

While the recovery process is a continual effort that takes place after one training session and into the next, you can get off to a good start by paying close attention to what you consume immediately and within the two hours after exercise. Then follow these post-exercise nutrition practices with food and fluid choices that match your daily training requirements.

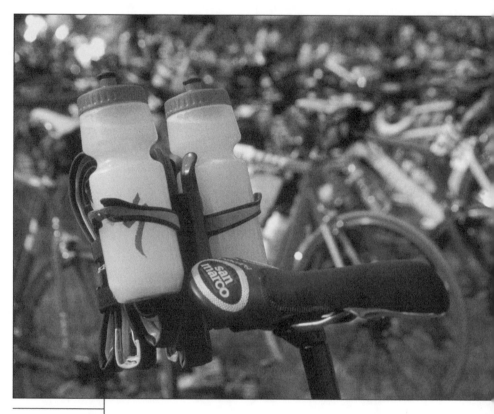

TOM MORAN PHOTO

chapter 5

EATING FOR TRAINING AND COMPETITION

Timing Matters

NUTRITION BEFORE TRAINING AND COMPETITION

Ideally you will consume a recovery diet designed to take you in top nutritional form from one cycling, running, or skiing session to the next. However, real life can sometimes (or perhaps often) get in the way of recharging your fuel stores to the optimal levels required for quality training. A hectic training schedule often leaves little leftover time for eating, let alone meal preparation. For some endurance athletes, multiple daily training sessions often result in brief windows of time during which the recommended amount of fuels must be quickly consumed. Yet paying attention to the foods you eat several days, twenty-four hours, and in the four-hour period before training and competition is worth the effort as these choices can significantly impact the quality of your athletic performance.

Because you are an endurance athlete, the longer and harder your training session is, the greater the risk of developing glycogen depletion and dehydration. Remember that your full supply of glycogen stores provide anywhere from 1,400 to 1,800 calories of fuel. At moderate to high intensities, you can cycle, run, and swim through these fuel stores in one to three hours. Once you experience muscle glycogen depletion, fatigue will set in as you "hit the wall." Even with plenty of fat stores still remaining, you may need to decrease your exercise intensity or you may not even be able to complete the training session. Your fat stores cannot supply fuel quickly enough, and consequently your muscle fibers don't receive the fuel needed to contract during exercise.

Blood glucose, maintained by your liver glycogen stores, is also your brain's only fuel source. When you run low on blood glucose, or "bonk," you cannot focus on the exercise task at hand. You may experience light-headedness, poor concentration, irritability, and even become disoriented during exercise. Exercise will seem much harder, and coordination and judgment will suffer. Your judgment may become impaired and affect your cycling technique off-road or in a pack, your skills may suffer while skiing, or you may have difficulty navigating your trail run. You may also have to slow down considerably or stop exercise altogether, as the blood glucose supplied by your liver is also an important fuel source for your muscles when they become depleted of glycogen.

While glycogen depletion can become a significant factor at moderate to high intensities and limit your training beyond one hour, other body nutrient stores may also become depleted. Fluid depletion or dehydration is also an important concern and can impede your training efforts. Depending on environmental conditions, the event, and the individual athlete, significant electrolyte depletion can also occur and stop your training in its tracks. Of particular concern, particularly for ultra-endurance events, is the development of depleted blood sodium or hyponatremia.

Endurance athletes who want to complete their training program or compete at their best would benefit from several nutrition strategies designed to minimize the fuel, fluid, and electrolyte depletion that can occur during endurance exercise. Making the most of specific food and fluid choices before training or competition offers several important performance advantages, such as:

- Beginning training or competition with optimal fluid levels to help delay or minimize dehydration.
- Refilling liver glycogen stores and decreasing risk of developing hypoglycemia during exercise.

- Topping off muscle glycogen stores and delaying glycogen depletion while training and competing.
- Providing fuel and fluid during the early part of exercise.
- Settling your stomach and preventing hunger pains during longer exercise sessions.
- Providing a psychological edge and comfort level, particularly during competition.

Clearly, stocking up on your liver and muscle glycogen stores before exercise is essential prior to endurance training. Nutritional strategies recommended before exercise vary depending on how close to training or competition you need to eat. Endurance athletes such as triathletes and marathon runners who compete several times yearly, peaking for specific races, can plan one week in advance to "carbohydrate load" their body fuel stores. Cyclists, on the other hand, may race every weekend and need to make the most of the four-hour period before competition to top off glycogen stores. And regardless of your chosen endurance sport, your training and work or school schedule often leaves you in the position of eating on the run, often in that four-hour period before exercise. Training, of course, is also your dress rehearsal for competition. Knowing what you tolerate and like right before training means that you will have ironed out these important details for the day of competition. Proper planning and eating ensures you have no unexpected surprises that result in coping with unpleasant gastrointestinal symptoms rather than performing your best on the race course.

One Week Prior to Competition—Carbohydrate Loading

When you have the luxury of tapering for an important competition event such as a triathlon, marathon, endurance ski event, adventure race, or swim competition, you are presented with the prime opportunity to maximize your carbohydrate fuel stores. The combination of not dipping into your muscle glycogen stores as deeply as you would with regular training and maximizing your carbohydrate intake is known as "carbohydrate loading." Traditionally considered to take place over a week, some athletes may also practice this strategy over a 24- to 48-hour period before competition. Research indicates that muscle glycogen stores return to normal with twenty-four hours of rest and a high carbohydrate diet if there is no significant muscle damage. However, it may be ideal to rest and eat up for an additional twenty-four hours to bring muscle glycogen levels from the normal full level of 100–120 millimoles per kilogram (mmol/kg) wet weight to the supercompensated level of 150–200 mmol/kg. Carbohydrate loading will allow you to run at your desired pace for a longer period of time and is especially useful for competition lasting longer than ninety minutes.

Sports nutritionists currently recommend the "modified" carbohydrate loading regimen that is gentler but just as effective as the old carbohydrate loading strategy that contained a stringent "depletion" phase. Devised in the 1960s, this depletion phase started a week before competition and lasted about three to four days. Glycogen stores were depleted with a combination of hard training and a low carbohydrate diet. This was followed by three to four days of combined rest and a high carbohydrate diet to glycogen-load the muscle. Athletes often complained of feeling and training poorly during the depletion phase, which occurred so close to competition.

This difficult depletion strategy was phased out after research in the 1980s demonstrated that it was unnecessary to achieve the desired high levels of muscle glycogen. Athletes were found to glycogen overload their muscles with a three- to four-day taper combined with a high carbohydrate diet. Below are a few guidelines to consider when carbohydrate loading:

- Gradually taper your training for one week prior to the event (longer if that is outlined in your training program). Eat your normal training diet during this one-week taper.
- For the last few days of the week, taper your training further or even rest completely for one to three days. Consume a high carbohydrate diet providing from

3 to 5 grams carbohydrates per pound weight. Your caloric needs may decrease during this time, but the proportion of carbohydrates in your diet should be increased.

- If you cannot taper for one week, reduce your training for three days and load up on carbohydrates.

- Exercise lightly the day before if needed to relieve any muscle stiffness and to keep your muscles "sharp" for competition.

- Have a food plan laid out ahead of time that ensures that you consume enough carbohydrates to glycogen load. Carbohydrate loading is not synonymous with "pigging out" and a food free-for-all. You don't want high fat foods to replace those precious carbohydrates.

- You may want to emphasize low fiber and compact carbohydrate food sources to minimize any gastrointestinal upset and to ensure that you consume the prescribed carbohydrate amounts.

- Be aware that for every gram of glycogen you store in your body, you also store up to three grams of water. This effect can result in a several pound weight gain. This extra fluid will help delay dehydration during the event.

- Pay close attention to what you eat the night before and the day of competition. Specific guidelines will be provided later in this chapter.

Having a sound menu plan in mind can take some of the stress off of carbohydrate loading. Table 5.1 provides a list of some high carbohydrate, low fiber foods that should be well tolerated in the several days before exercise and that provide 30 grams of carbohydrates per listed serving. Starches, breads, and cereals that are low in fiber are fairly concentrated sources. Fruit and fruit juices are also good sources of carbohydrates. And sports nutrition supplements such as energy bars, gels, concentrated carbohydrate drinks, and high carbohydrate meal replacements may also fit nicely into your meal plan.

The food lists in Chapter 6 provide you with an extended list of 30-gram carbohydrate servings. You may want to consider decreasing your intake of proteins and fats during this carbohydrate-loading phase so as not to shut out the carbohydrates required for full replenishment of stored fuel. Consuming between-meal snacks is another strategy for obtaining the recommended carbohydrate amounts. Buying some of the sports supplements and commercial products available may make life simpler and easier during carbohydrate loading. Table 5.2 provides a sample menu for a very high carbohydrate loading day at more than 700 grams of carbohydrate. If this level exceeds your carbohydrate needs, simply trim back on some of the carbohydrate portions or one or more of the listed snacks.

The Day before the Event

Often training sessions and competitions

5.1

PRE-EXERCISE HIGH CARBOHYDRATE, LOW FIBER FOODS

30 Grams of Carbohydrate Per Serving
Apple, 1.5 medium
Apple juice, 8 oz.
Applesauce, sweetened, 1/2 cup
Bagel, 2 oz.
Bread, white, 2 slices
Canned fruit, 1 cup
Carrot juice, 10 oz.
Cold cereal, low fiber, 1.5 oz.
Cooked cereal, 1 cup
Cranberry juice cocktail, 8 oz.
Dinner rolls, 2
English muffin, 1
Graham crackers, 6
Grape juice, 6 oz.
Grapefruit, peeled, 1 large
Milk, skim, 20 oz.
Muffin, low fat, low fiber, 3 oz.
Pasta, cooked, 1 cup
Pita pocket, 1.5 rounds
Potato, baked, no skin, 1 medium
Pretzels, white flour, 1.5 oz.
Rice, cooked, white, 2/3 cup
Saltines, 8
Sweet potato, no skin, 4 oz.
Tortillas, 2
Yogurt with fruit, 1 cup

take place in the early morning after liver glycogen stores become 80 percent depleted from the overnight fast. Because liver glycogen is an important source of blood glucose during exercise, exercising in this fasted state can cause an unwanted drop in blood glucose. Having a high carbohydrate dinner and perhaps even a light snack high in carbohydrates will fill your liver with glycogen the night before, somewhat diminishing the effect of low morning liver glycogen. Just make sure that any late-night noshes are easy to digest. The day before and especially the night before the event you do not want to try any new and unusual foods that could result in gastrointestinal upset. Go to bed comfortably full, not stuffed. Avoid consuming large

5.2

SAMPLE CARBO-LOADING ONE-DAY MENU

Breakfast
Orange juice, 1 cup
Cornflakes, 2 cups
Banana, 1 large
Skim milk, 1 cup
Toast, 2 slices
Margarine, 1 tsp.
Jelly, 2 Tbsp.
147 g carbohydrates, 895 calories

Snack
Yogurt with fruit, 1 cup
45 g carbohydrates, 240 calories

Lunch
Lean turkey, 3 oz.
White bread, 2 slices
Pretzels, 1 1/2 oz.
Pear, 1 large
Apple juice, 12 oz.
135 g carbohydrates, 725 calories

Snack
Energy bar
Liquid supplement, 12–16 oz.
135 g carbohydrates, 1,040 calories

Dinner
Rice, cooked, 2 cups
Ground turkey, 3 oz.
Peas, cooked, 1 cup
Bread, 2 slices
160 g carbohydrates, 961 calories

Snack
Frozen yogurt, 12 oz.
Fig newtons, 2
102 g carbohydrates, 460 calories

Total: 724 g carbohydrates, 4,321 calories

amounts of protein and fat, which take longer to digest and could push out carbohydrates. Be especially careful to limit fiber-containing foods, gassy foods such as broccoli and beans, and avoid alcohol. Practice having various meals the night before an important morning training session. Make simple meals that can be ordered in most restaurants when traveling. Pasta dishes low in fat (no Alfredo, please) are a common favorite among athletes, but other choices also work well. Try rice based dishes, stir-fried noodles, baked potatoes, and load up on white breads. You probably want to avoid salads and other raw vegetables and raw fruits the night before an important training session or race.

The Day of the Event

Three to Four Hours before Exercise

Depending on your race time, personal tolerances, and experience, you should consume a light to large meal in the three to four hours before competition. Many seasoned endurance athletes have identified this time interval as optimal for pre-exercise or pre-race eating, as you can achieve a good balance between optimal food consumption and adequate digestion time. Hopefully you will greet the morning well hydrated and with muscle glycogen stored at peak levels by practicing the proper nutrition techniques several days before the race. The main focus of this pre-race meal should be to replenish your liver glycogen stores. This valuable fuel falls to low levels overnight, especially if you spent your sleep tossing and turning from pre-race nerves. With the right timing and portions, eating three to four hours before exercise will allow you to:

- Restore liver glycogen to normal levels.
- Store carbohydrates in the muscle as needed if portions are large enough.
- Have some carbohydrates stored in the gut for absorption and release during exercise.
- Avoid feeling hungry during longer events.

The morning of competition it is especially important to choose foods that you enjoy and tolerate and that also provide both a physiological and psychological edge. For every hour you allow yourself to digest, consume just less than half a gram of carbohydrates for every pound that you weigh. For example, if you decide to eat a larger meal four hours before a triathlon or swim competition, you can consume two grams of carbohydrates per pound weight. For a 150-pound athlete this translates to 300 grams of carbohydrates (and 1,200 calories). It would probably be easiest on your stomach if a good portion of this fairly substantial meal consisted of dense low fiber foods and some liquid carbohydrate sources. You can obtain 300 grams of carbohydrates by consuming one large bagel topped with two tablespoons of jam, followed by a fruited yogurt and 32 ounces of a concentrated sports drink. The small amounts of protein in the yogurt may help keep you full a bit longer. You can also add peanut butter or cream cheese to your bagel if a small amount of fat is well tolerated. Of course smaller meals may be only what some athletes tolerate close to exercise, particularly competition. Every athlete needs to iron out individual tolerances in terms of foods, portions, and timing.

PRE-EXERCISE, HIGH CARBOHYDRATE, LOW FAT MEALS

Toast or small bagel, 2 slices Banana, 1 large Jelly, 2 Tbsp. Juice, 8 oz. **120 g carbohydrates** **520 calories**	Concentrated carbohydrate beverage, 1.5 cups Toast, 1 slice **90 g carbohydrates** **380 calories**	Carbohydrate gel, 1 serving Sports drink, 24 oz. **95 g carbohydrates** **380 calories**
Chicken, 2 oz. Bread, 2 slices Fruit juice, 16 oz. Pretzels, 2 oz. Carbohydrate supplement, 16 oz. **220 g carbohydrates** **1,030 calories**	Pasta, cooked, 2 cups Marinara sauce, 1 cup Bread, 2 slices Frozen yogurt, 12 oz. Fruit juice, 8 oz. Margarine, 2 tsp. **235 g carbohydrates** **986 calories**	Pancakes, 4 medium Fruit topping, 1/2 cup Syrup, 1/2 cup Fruit juice, 8 oz. **270 g carbohydrates** **1,200 calories**

Cooked cereal, 2 cups
Instant breakfast drink,
  1 serving
Banana, 1 large
Orange juice, 8 oz.
Carbohydrate beverage,
  24 oz.
 	
300 g carbohydrates
1,410 calories
	Rice, cooked, 3 cups
	Cooked vegetables, 1 cup
	Shrimp, 4 oz.
	Sorbet, 1 cup
	Soft drink, 12 oz.
	Oil, 2 tsp.
	Carbohydrate beverage,
	  16 oz.
	
	300 g carbohydrates
	1,600 calories
		Fruit smoothie:
		  Yogurt, 8 oz.
		  Milk, 8 oz.
		  Juice, 8 oz.
		  1 cup fruit
		
		Bagel, 1 large
		Jam, 2 Tbsp.
		Energy bar, 1 whole
		
		225 g carbohydrates
		1,185 calories

Eating three to four hours before exercise is an often-favored pre-exercise meal timing that can be very appropriate for several exercise start times. Typically, you may want to rise early and eat for a morning start (some athletes even get up to eat and go back to sleep). This timing interval also allows for a hefty mid-morning meal prior to an afternoon start time. Table 5.3 provides some examples of pre-exercise meals. Clearly, reaching more than 200 grams of carbohydrates in a meal requires planning, some high carbohydrate supplements, and a strong stomach!

Two Hours before Exercise

Consuming food three to four hours before exercise may not always be possible due to scheduling and very early morning start times (rising at 3:00 a.m. to eat does not sound very appealing). Because of timing constraints, eating two hours before training and competition may be your preferred timing. One solid food rule for pre-exercise eating is the closer to exercise you plan to eat, the smaller the meal consumed. Try to keep your intake of carbohydrates to one gram per pound of body weight in this time interval. A 150-pound athlete could consume 150 grams of carbohydrates or less. With this close meal timing, it likely is even more important that liquid choices beef up your meal. Breakfast shakes, liquid meal replacements, and sports supplements often provide more than 50 grams of carbohydrates per serving. A juice smoothie may work well, as do easily digested energy bars.

Eating two hours prior to exercise could be good timing for an early or mid-morning start. It can also work well for tricky early afternoon start times. Follow a large breakfast that is well-digested with a small snack two hours before exercise to provide fuel and prevent hunger during competition and training.

Eating an Hour before Exercise—Separating Fact from Fallacy

There are a variety of scenarios that could necessitate the need for food thirty to sixty minutes prior to exercise. Rising in the extremely early hours of the morning simply to eat food and fuel up for an early start time may not be feasible or desirable. Scheduling may also result in a long time gap between the last meal and the start of a training session, and hunger and limited fuel during training and competition may become a significant issue. It may also be helpful to eat closer to longer training sessions in which the added fuel provides a performance benefit. Despite these practical considerations, consuming carbohydrates in the hour prior to exercise has been a subject of some controversy over the years.

It began in 1979 when a well-respected lab reported the results of one preliminary study. When subjects were fed 75 grams of glucose thirty to forty-five minutes prior to exercise, the researchers measured a decrease in blood glucose levels, or hypoglycemia, during exercise. An exercise test also measured a decrease in performance at 80 percent VO_2 max when compared to a placebo. However, what was not as widely reported from this study was that the measured hypoglycemia was short-lived, lasting only about ten minutes into exercise, and was not associated with fatigue during exercise.

These results spurred more research. Nine studies had subjects consume a variety of supplemental carbohydrate sources such as fructose, glucose, sucrose, and amylopectin in supplement form (rather than from real food) anywhere from thirty to sixty minutes prior to exercise. Five of these studies found that the carbohydrate feeding did not impair exercise, while four of these studies found an actual performance improvement. So overall, eating thirty to sixty minutes prior to exercise is very unlikely to impair performance and may even provide a needed performance boost. But what was most interesting about the study results was the highly individual metabolic responses among subjects, with some subjects (a small number) experiencing hypoglycemia.

Because some athletes do experience more symptomatic transient hypoglycemia than others, subsequent research studies incorporated the glycemic index (GI) into their study design. As previously mentioned, lower glycemic index foods produce more stable blood glucose and lower insulin responses than moderate or high GI foods. It was thought that consuming a lower glycemic index food would be better tolerated thirty to sixty minutes prior to exercise and could improve performance. In other words, a bowl of home cooked oats, rather than a big glob of carbohydrate gel, may give you a more sustained boost when skiing.

When low glycemic foods were incorporated into several types of study designs, results for nine studies were split down the middle. Utilizing a lower GI food did appear to lessen the observation of marked responses in insulin and lowering of blood glucose levels. However, the performance implications of this manipulated metabolic response were less clear. Some studies found an improvement in performance, while others did not. And it appears that the best designed studies (which directly compared a low glycemic food to a high glycemic food) found no performance improvement with the low glycemic food despite the blood glucose response being favorably altered.

From an athlete's perspective, whether or not you consume carbohydrates thirty to sixty minutes prior to exercise needs to be individualized to your tolerances and training or competition schedule. Deriving a performance benefit from ingesting fuel thirty to sixty minutes prior to exercise is most likely to occur when the carbohydrates you consume replenish compromised fuel stores. So consider consuming carbohydrates within an hour before exercise if you have not eaten for four hours or more, or prior to early morning training when liver glycogen is low. Eating before long training sessions can also prevent hunger and would provide extra calories for triathletes, skiers, marathon runners, and other endurance athletes who have very high energy requirements.

If you are still concerned that you are carbohydrate sensitive during the hour prior to exercise, there are a few sensible strategies that you may find useful. Consuming a high enough amount of carbohydrates may simply offset any lowered blood glucose levels and hypoglycemic symptoms. Amounts of 70 grams or more seem to maintain blood glucose levels in individuals susceptible to exercise hypoglycemia. Individuals not susceptible to hypoglycemia can consume anywhere from 50 to 100 grams of carbohydrates prior to exercise depending on what they prefer and what feels comfortable. You can also consider a carbohydrate source with a lower glycemic index, though this often requires the consumption of real foods very close to exercise rather than easily digested sports nutrition products. Common sense would indicate that consuming a carbohydrate beverage or gel might be more practical than chowing down on a big bowl of lentils the hour before exercise. Many products such as gels, bars, and sports drinks provide anywhere from 30 to 50 grams of carbohydrates per serving. You may choose one of the items or any combination of them in portions that you tolerate.

Regardless of your start time, a pre-competition (or pre-training) meal or snack can provide some performance benefit. While the main part of your intake will be carbohydrates, small amounts of protein and perhaps fat may be tolerated if appropriately timed. Determine your optimal pre-exercise meal through experimentation during training, not on race day. Table 5.4 reviews some pre-exercise meal timing strategies.

Timing and Portions

The bottom line is that you should focus on pre-race or pre-training nutrition that is appropriate for your competitive event and training schedule. If you taper for a competition, carbohydrate loading provides the opportune strategy that results in muscle glycogen stores that are slightly above normal levels. The morning of the race, you can decide on the pre-race meal timing that best suits your preferences and tolerances. Specific amounts of carbohydrates consumed at set times prior to exercise have been shown to enhance performance by increasing liver glycogen stores and providing fuel during the early part of exercise. Athletes who feel that they are sensitive to consuming carbohydrates in the hour before exercise can make sure that they ingest more than 70 grams of carbohydrates to offset any hypoglycemia.

Hydration before Exercise

Dehydration is one of the most significant problems that occurs during endurance exercise, and it can put a halt to your training long before glycogen depletion will stop you in your tracks. Despite your best attempts to drink adequately during exercise, you are unlikely to match 100 percent of your fluid losses. Significant dehydration can especially occur in athletes who have very high sweat rates, when there is little opportunity to drink while you train, or when environmental conditions are extreme.

Just as strategies to maximize muscle glycogen stores are appealing, so are techniques for maximizing fluid stores before exercise. But hyperhydrating is not considered to be as optimal as drinking during exercise to replace fluid losses, and the

HOW TO EAT BEFORE TRAINING AND COMPETITION

TIMING	START TIMES	CARBOHYDRATE/ FOOD RECOMMENDATIONS	SAMPLE FOODS
Night before	Essential for early starts Helpful for any start time	High carbohydrate meal 300 grams carbohydrate Low in fiber Plenty of fluid	Pasta dishes Rice dishes Lean protein Easy on fat Cooked vegetables
3–4 hours prior	**For Mid-morning start:** Eat at 7 a.m. for 10 a.m. start **For Mid-afternoon start:** Eat at 10 a.m. for 2 p.m. start	Carbohydrates: 1.5–2.0 g/lb. wt. (3.0–4.0 g/kg) Low fat proteins Low fat Low fiber Plenty of fluids	150-pound athlete: 225–300 g of carbohydrate Cereals, bread, crackers, milk, yogurt, fruit, juices, jelly, muffins, bagels
2 hours prior	**For Mid-morning start:** Eat at 8 a.m. for 10 a.m. start **For Mid-afternoon start:** Eat at 12 noon for 2 p.m. start after a large morning breakfast **For Late start:** Eat at 6 p.m. for 8 p.m. start after adequate carbohydrate meals throughout the day	Carbohydrates: Up to 1.0 g/lb. wt. (2.0 g/kg) Minimal low fat protein Low fat and fiber Plenty of fluids	150-pound athlete: 130–150 g carbohydrates Cereals, bread, milk, yogurt, fruit, juices, jelly, crackers
1 hour prior	**For Early start:** Eat at 6 a.m. for 8 a.m. start **For Mid-morning start:** For 10 a.m. start, have snack/liquid at 9 a.m. in addition to 6:30–7 a.m. meal	Carbohydrates: 0.5 g/lb. wt. (1.0 g/kg) Emphasize liquids Easy to digest carbohydrates Avoid protein, fat, and fiber	Sports drinks, concentrated carbohydrate drinks and gels, sports bars, tolerated fruits
Immediately prior	For any start time	Carbohydrates	Sports drinks Energy bars (if exercise starts at moderate intensity for at least 30 minutes)

physiological benefits of this strategy remain controversial. However, if you anticipate that it will be difficult to drink when you train or race due to limited fluid availability and race strategy, hyperhydrating could be a practical move on your part. Even the "best" drinkers typically replace only about 80 percent of sweat losses, and catch-up drinking is not an effective hydration strategy on hot days when you need to complete a long ride or run.

At all costs, avoid starting training or competition in a dehydrated state and rendering any future drinking efforts to the futile and often ill-tolerated realm of catch-up drinking. As previously mentioned, one of the best gauges of your hydration efforts during exercise is to weigh yourself before and after training. Every pound of weight loss represents 16 ounces of fluid loss. However, to compensate for urine losses when rehydrating, you should consume 24 ounces of fluid for every pound decrease in weight. Techniques for drinking more during exercise will be discussed later in this chapter.

It is important to plan ahead and begin your next training session as well hydrated as possible. To prepare for the next day's training, consume 16 ounces of fluid before bedtime. Your early morning intake should then consist of 16–24 ounces of mainly caffeine free fluid. Caffeine-containing fluids should be kept to moderate levels. Prior to training, you should attempt to consume 8–10 ounces of fluid every hour during the day. About one hour before exercise you can hyperhydrate by consuming 16–32 ounces of fluid. At this time, fluids providing carbohydrates and small amounts of sodium, such as sports drinks, are likely to be the best choice and may have some hydration advantages over water. You can fill your fluid stores further by drinking another 8–16 ounces, twenty minutes prior to training. Similar guidelines can be followed prior to competition, although you will want to time bathroom break opportunities carefully. Prior to competition, you may decide to stop drinking thirty minutes prior to the race. This strategy should allow you to empty your bladder if needed and not compromise your hydration status if you have consumed adequate fluid in the hours prior to the race.

Priming your stomach immediately before exercise with a fluid load is a useful strategy if tolerated. The rate at which fluid leaves your stomach and enters your small intestine for absorption is slightly increased when the stomach is stretched. Experiment to see what volumes do not exceed your comfort level. It is best to practice these fluid-intake guidelines prior to training, not competition.

In summary, you will be adequately hydrated if you focus on these simple guidelines:

- Consume 16 ounces of fluid before bedtime.
- Consume 8–10 ounces of fluid during the day when not training.
- Hyperhydrate one hour before exercise by consuming 16–32 ounces of fluid.
- Consume another 8–16 ounces, twenty minutes prior to exercise if possible.

NUTRITION DURING TRAINING AND COMPETITION

Fluid Requirements

While an Ironman triathlon and other ultraendurance events can represent the extreme in heat related fluid and electrolyte losses, staying well hydrated and fueled during training and competition can enhance any endurance exercise effort. The longer and harder you exercise, the greater the risk that nutrient losses can impair your performance. That's why consuming adequate fluid, carbohydrates, and electrolytes during competition is beneficial. This practice can:

- Prevent dehydration.
- Maintain blood glucose levels.
- Offset muscle and liver glycogen depletion.
- Fuel your brain and prevent central nervous system fatigue.

Moderate to high intensity exercise of longer duration is the activity most likely to result in dehydration. One study found a 34-percent decrease in maximum cycling time with only a 2-percent drop in body weight due to dehydration. Increased muscle temperature also leads to premature glycogen depletion and can cut your planned training program short. There are many good reasons for preventing dehydration. The physiological effects of dehydration include:

- Increased heart rate
- Increased body temperature
- Decreased blood volume
- Increased perception of effort
- Compromised mental concentration
- Compromised fine motor skills
- Delayed stomach emptying of fluids
- Increased risk of gastrointestinal upset

While average sweat losses are 1–1.5 quarts per hour, losses can reach 2–3 quarts per hour during hot weather and high intensity exercise. Sweat rates not only vary with environmental conditions, but vary greatly among athletes. A high level of fitness also promotes a more efficient sweat response. The better trained you are the more you will sweat.

While your ideal goal is to match your fluid intake to your fluid losses, most athletes fall short and replace only 50 to 80 percent of their fluid losses during exercise. Even with strong efforts to match your fluid losses, your gastrointestinal system may only be able to absorb a certain amount of fluid at one time. Often, whether or not you can maintain full hydration status during exercise is a matter of practicality rather than scientific theory. Consuming the recommended amounts can be challenging due to logistics, limited opportunities to drink, availability of fluids, taste preferences, and gastrointestinal tolerances.

Clearly you need to assess the situation for your own sport, whether cycling and carrying fluids, or swimming and placing fluids at the end of your lane, and plan accordingly. Many endurance athletes do carry their own fluid and food supplies during exercise in some fashion, while others rely heavily on aid stations, helpful team personnel, or friends. Regardless of how they reach you, you are more likely

Traveling for Competition

It is important to consider how travel affects your pre-competition nutrition program and plan accordingly. Special meals can be ordered on airlines with advance notice. Try to bring your own 1- to 2-quart bottle of fluid on board to maintain adequate hydration levels. Make smart choices at the airport. Aim for turkey sandwiches or wraps, frozen yogurt, fruit juice, fresh fruit, soft pretzels, baked potatoes, milk, and smoothies. Plan ahead and pack some of your favorite non-perishable items such energy bars, granola bars, cereals, packets of instant breakfast mix, dried fruit, cereals, crackers, powdered sports drinks, meal replacements, instant soups, fruit juice, and any items that travel safely.

You can also investigate the food options at your destination before you leave. Call ahead to your accommodations and find out about food establishments in your area, especially if traveling internationally. Speak with individuals who have competed at your destination in the past. If food safety issues in a foreign country are a concern, restrict yourself to bottled water and well-cooked foods and avoid high-risk foods such as ice cubes and unpeeled fruits and vegetables. Better safe than sorry. ■

to consume fluids that taste good and that are the right temperature. Commercial sports drinks often appeal to hot, sweaty athletes. In addition to their flavor, which may stimulate you to drink more, sports drinks are a source of fuel and electrolytes in the form of carbohydrates and sodium chloride. Below are some hydration strategies designed to maximize your fluid intake during exercise:

Consume 4–8 ounces of fluid every 15 to 20 minutes of exercise. Practice, practice, practice. Set your heart rate monitor or watch to remind you to drink at specific intervals. Try to take big gulps, as larger volumes empty from your stomach more quickly. Cooler fluids empty from your stomach more quickly as well.

Start drinking early. Even if you start exercise adequately hydrated, it does not pay to practice catch-up drinking. Once you are dehydrated, fluids will empty from your stomach more slowly. In extreme situations dehydration may lead to GI upset including a bloated stomach and vomiting. Because fluids are emptying slowly, you will feel dehydrated (you *are* dehydrated) and compensate by drinking more, further aggravating any GI intolerance.

Monitor your sweat rates during training. It is important that you appreciate the rate at which you lose fluid during varying training sessions and environmental conditions. Practice drinking during race-like conditions. Monitor your weight before and after exercise to assess how effectively you replace fluids.

Develop a taste for various sports drinks. While you may discover your favorite sports drink brand and flavor to use during training, this product may not always be available to you during competition. Some competitive events may permit carrying of your favorite products, but you may also be limited to what is available on the course. Find out what product will be served at important competitions, and get accustomed to its taste and feel during training. This allows for greater flexibility and improved drinking during race day.

Fuel Requirements

Research from dozens of studies has clearly demonstrated that carbohydrate intake during exercise of greater than ninety minutes and at moderate intensity is performance enhancing. Carbohydrates consumed during exercise can maintain blood glucose levels and provide fuel to glycogen-depleted muscles. Carbohydrate consumption may also provide the opportunity for glucose to be stored in less active muscle fibers. For example, when you train at a low intensity, muscle fibers that fuel higher intensity efforts may be replenished. This may explain why some endurance athletes are able to dig deep and sprint to the finish after a long bout of challenging racing. Another important effect of consuming carbohydrates during exercise is to spare liver glycogen, allowing the liver to maintain glucose output later in exercise.

Your brain may also benefit from carbohydrate intake during long training runs or rides. It has been measured that consuming only water during endurance exercise will decrease blood glucose levels. Because your brain counts on glucose for fuel, this will result in some negative central nervous system effects. Carbohydrates can prevent or reverse symptoms of glucose deprivation such as fatigue, perception of increased effort, and poor coordination. Carbohydrates are also thought to prevent an increase in brain serotonin levels that can occur during prolonged exercise. Serotonin produces feelings of drowsiness and fatigue in the brain.

Besides fueling your brain and providing performance benefits for exercise lasting about ninety minutes, carbohydrates may also improve performance during high intensity exercise lasting about sixty minutes. Several studies over the past decade measured the performance effects of consuming a sports drink during exercise performed at 80 to 90 percent VO_2 max and lasting about one hour. Results indicated that the sports drink provided a performance benefit. Several additional studies measured the performance effects upon intermittent high intensity exercise lasting about one hour. Consuming a sports drink at rest intervals allowed the activity to continue longer. Researchers speculated that the carbohydrate drinks provided the fast-twitch muscle fibers, which operate at higher intensities, some fuel to work with at rest intervals between high intensity efforts.

More research measuring the effects of carbohydrate consumption on exercise lasting one hour is needed. It has also yet to be determined what effect carbohydrate consumption has on exercise lasting less than one hour. Consumption of carbohydrates during shorter endurance efforts (sixty to ninety minutes) may also be a viable alternative if you arrive to the training session with less than optimal carbohydrate stores due to a hectic schedule and other challenges that get in the way of optimal food intake. Carbohydrate consumption may also be worth testing during interval training, as it may allow you to train at these intermittent higher intensities for longer.

Sports Drinks

Clearly, both fluid and carbohydrates are required during endurance exercise and very possibly during high intensity exercise lasting one hour and during interval training. In order for your body to receive both carbohydrates and fluid in a timely and well-tolerated manner, several steps in the digestion and absorption of sports drinks must be considered. First, when you consume these nutrients they must empty as quickly as possible from your stomach. Next, they then enter your small intestine where they must be absorbed as quickly as possible and then enter the bloodstream. Carbohydrates are then available as fuel for your exercising muscles.

In an effort to provide the most scientifically sound formulation, sports drink research has looked at each one of these steps to see where the flow may actually slow down or speed up. If your sports drink gets bogged down in any one of the steps, that means it takes the fluid and carbohydrates that much longer to reach you. Consequently, the sports drink is not as performance enhancing. It has been determined that the two factors that determine how quickly a sports drink leaves your stomach are the volume of fluid in your stomach and the concentration of the carbohydrates in the drink.

Concentration

The greater the concentration of the fluid, the longer it takes to leave your stomach. What research has determined is that carbohydrate solutions of about 4 to 8 percent concentration empty from your stomach very efficiently. Conveniently, most sports drinks fall into this gastrically acceptable range (about 6 to 8 percent carbohydrate).

Solutions falling into this range deliver an optimal balance of both carbohydrates and fluid. This drink concentration allows fluid to reach your bloodstream pretty much as quickly as water, but still delivers performance boosting carbohydrates at an acceptable rate. Drinks of these concentrations are also well tolerated by most athletes. Tolerance to these products can also improve with practice. In contrast, drinks of 10 to 12 percent concentration, such as soft drinks, are emptied more slowly and are not as hydrating. Drinks of less than 4 percent concentration would not supply enough carbohydrates to enhance performance, but would still be hydrating.

Volume

As mentioned previously, volume affects the degree of stomach distention and consequently affects gastric emptying. Increased stomach distention will result in liquids emptying from your stomach more quickly, with about 50 percent of stomach contents being emptied every ten minutes. To maximize emptying, try to start exercise with a comfortably full stomach and drink at regular intervals of about 10 to 15 minutes if possible. How much fluid an athlete can empty from the stomach is highly variable. However, emptying rates of 24–40 ounces or 3–5 cups per hour are commonly seen.

Intestinal Absorption

Studies measuring intestinal absorption rates have determined that sports drink solutions are as readily absorbed as water. Different forms of carbohydrates are absorbed across the intestinal wall, utilizing various transport mechanisms. Again, higher concentration drinks should be avoided, as they draw water into the intestinal tract before being absorbed.

The wide variety of sports drink products available also provides a wide variety of carbohydrate sources. These include glucose polymers, glucose, sucrose, and fructose. Many drinks have a mix, allowing various carbohydrate types to be transported simultaneously. These carbohydrate mixes all appear to have a moderate to high glycemic index—handy for quickly raising blood glucose levels—and give you a quick burst of both brain power and energy when consumed. Glucose polymers do not seem to offer any absorption advantages over glucose, but are popular because they have a milder rather than overly sweet taste. Fructose is the only beverage not used in high amounts or solely in a sports beverage. Large amounts of fructose are not well absorbed and can lead to GI upset. But drinks that contain some fructose should provide easily tolerated concentrations and additional flavor.

Quantity and Timing of Carbohydrate Consumption

Basically the amounts of sports drinks you consume should mimic the water intake guidelines described previously, or about 4–8 ounces every fifteen to twenty minutes. Performance benefits begin when about 30 grams of carbohydrates per hour are delivered. However, 50–60 grams may be optimal to meet fuel needs during exercise after muscle glycogen depletion has occurred. Every athlete has his or her own personal tolerances and carbohydrate requirements that maintain optimal energy levels during exercise. Some athletes competing in ultraendurance events may consume up to 100 grams of carbohydrates per hour not only from sports drinks, but other carbohydrate options as well.

When relying solely on a sports drink for replacing carbohydrate losses, you would have to consume 32 ounces of a 6-percent solution in one hour to obtain 60 grams of carbohydrate. A 7-percent solution provides 50 grams when 24 ounces is consumed in one hour. Check labels and instructions of your favorite sports drinks. Then determine how much you would need to consume in one hour to obtain 30–60 grams of carbohydrate. Experiment to determine what fluid consumption best enhances your performance.

As far as timing is concerned, large single feedings and smaller, regular intakes of a sports drink are both beneficial. Basically, drink whenever possible given the nature of the training session and competition. Steady state exercise, such as a downhill section of a ski race or when cycling at moderate intensity in a pack, provides the best opportunity to drink. Consuming carbohydrate after depletion has set in can help, but consuming the carbohydrates early on in order to prevent fatigue is prudent. Don't wait until the signs and symptoms of a low fuel tank register before consuming your carbohydrate beverage.

Form of Carbohydrate

Liquid, semi-liquid, and solid carbohydrates are well tolerated by many athletes during exercise, though these tolerances can vary. Obviously, carbohydrate drinks offer the advantage of hydration and fuel. While sports drinks are practical, many endurance athletes like using some of the more concentrated carbohydrate gels for situations when energy needs outweigh the desire for fluid. These products, however, should be consumed with some fluid. More solid items such as energy bars, bananas, or fig newtons are also well tolerated by many endurance athletes such as cyclists who experience minimal stomach jostling. Often these foods take some of the edge off hunger during a long ski session or mountain bike ride. Endurance athletes can also learn to tolerate beverages of a more concentrated nature, with a common example being liquid meals consumed during competitions such as long road cycling stages. These products help offset the very high fuel demands of the exercise.

Basically fluid and carbohydrate choices can be somewhat individualized. Sometimes it is possible for fluid needs to be of greater significance, as on a hot, humid day, so a 4-percent concentration that is not overly sweet and thirst-quenching may be desired. If carbohydrate needs are a greater priority, such as later on in exercise, gels, bars, and more concentrated carbohydrate fluids that provide a shot of energy may be emphasized.

Usually a range of nutritional choices is ingested over the course of an endurance event, and you should fine-tune your balance of meeting both energy and fluid needs while considering your GI tolerances. Sometimes the pace of exercise may need to be adjusted to accommodate nutritional intake, or athletes can take advantage of lulls in the pace. Usually these adjustments are offset by the performance benefits derived from maintaining an appropriate nutritional intake.

The Electrolyte Edge

Though sweat is mainly water, it does contain a number of electrolytes. However, the concentration of these electrolytes in sweat is much lower than that found in body fluids. Composition of sweat can also vary among athletes, mostly in regards to salt content. But because electrolytes are the major solid component of sweat, research has focused on replacement needs of these nutrients. Sodium and potassium have been most frequently studied, though chloride is also a consideration.

The major electrolytes lost in sweat are sodium and chloride, which form salt. You may have noticed dried salt on your body after heavy sweating. Minerals lost in small amounts from sweat include potassium, magnesium, calcium, iron, copper, and zinc. To appreciate if and when electrolyte replacement is required during exercise, you need to know what happens to blood electrolyte concentrations during exercise. During high sweat rates, the concentrations of sodium and potassium increase, chloride and calcium remain constant, and magnesium levels usually fall.

Overall, even during most prolonged exercise, electrolyte deficiencies probably won't occur. However, electrolyte imbalances may occur during ultraendurance events such as ultramarathons, adventure races, and Ironman triathlons. The recovery period after excessive sweating may also result in electrolyte deficiency. Minor sodium, chloride, and potassium losses need to be replaced daily with a balanced diet to prevent deficiencies from occurring over time. If losses are not replaced, a deficit may occur over four to seven days of hard training.

Generally, electrolyte replacement for most forms of exercise is not required. But the sodium found in sports drinks does improve taste and facilitate fluid and glucose absorption through the intestine. Sodium may also stimulate your thirst and drinking mechanism. The amount of sodium in most sports drinks is relatively low. These small amounts certainly are not detrimental to performance, while excessive intakes of salt may aggravate electrolyte balance.

However, during ultraendurance activity, cases of hyponatremia or low blood sodium have been identified. The most common cause of this potentially dangerous condition is likely overhydration that leads to water intoxication. During exercise lasting four to five hours or longer, athletes lose sodium through sweating, then consume large amounts of fluid, especially plain water. This fluid is retained, body fluids eventually become very diluted, and sodium levels decrease. Therefore, in ultraendurance events, solutions with a higher sodium content are recommended. Aim for 250–500 milligrams per hour. Some individual athletes may even lose 1,000 milligrams or more of sodium per hour from sweating, Specific sports drinks and gels are higher in sodium than others. A common practice among endurance athletes has become to consume low dose salt tablets with plenty of water. Athletes competing in these events can also increase their salt intake several days prior to racing to assure that blood sodium levels area at the high end of normal at start time. This ensures that any drops still leave blood sodium levels within the normal range. Depending on your event, you can plan some higher sodium foods and supplements into your race nutrition program. Consider adding some salt to your drinks as needed, but only after experimentation during training.

It can be difficult to identify athletes who are at greater risk for hyponatremia than others. Clearly the event needs to be several hours in length. It is not expected that the world's top marathoners are at risk for developing hyponatremia, as their race times are simply too short! It takes time to consume large amounts of fluid and thereby reduce your blood sodium levels. Athletes who are competing at higher intensities are also likely to find drinking fluids less convenient than a middle of the pack finisher.

While ongoing study will determine more about the risks of developing hyponatremia, what is emerging, as this condition receives more attention and study from medical team personnel and researchers, is that the slower finishers seem to be at greater risk for developing this potentially dangerous condition. Having a longer finish time simply provides a greater opportunity to drink more sodium-free fluid, and consequently to dilute your blood sodium levels. Endurance athletes should anticipate their finish times and plan accordingly. Have higher sodium beverages available for consumption during competition and increase salt intake several days before the race. You can also consider carrying salt tablets with you and consume them during the race.

Obtaining adequate fuel and fluid during exercise takes practice, experience, and experimentation. Below are some practical tips for making the most of your fluid and food intake during exercise.

Drink on a schedule and have a plan. Set your watch or heart rate monitor to remind you to drink. Check your intake every hour to determine if you are keeping up with the required fluid amounts.

Start exercise with a comfortably full stomach. This will speed up gastric emptying, as will drinking fluid every fifteen to twenty minutes.

Use a sports drink during high intensity exercise lasting sixty minutes and moderate to high intensity exercise lasting greater than ninety minutes. Research indicates that this combination of fluid and carbohydrates improves performance.

Consume 30–60 grams carbohydrates per hour from a sports drink. This amount will ensure that you do not become dehydrated and provide fuel as glycogen stores become depleted. Most sports drinks provide 14–20 grams of carbohydrates per 8-ounce serving. One full water bottle would provide 35–50 grams and should be consumed per hour of exercise.

Start drinking early on during exercise. Minimizing a fluid deficit makes more sense than reversing dehydration during exercise. Your brain also derives benefits from the carbohydrates consumed, and the carbohydrate spares liver glycogen stores that can be broken down for use later in exercise.

Experiment with other sources of carbohydrates. During longer events a more solid form of carbohydrates may be appealing and help mitigate hunger pains. Gels are semi-solid and provide up to 50 grams of carbohydrates per gulp. Just remember to consume gels with plenty of water; otherwise they will sit in your stomach, as they are a concentrated carbohydrate source. Solid foods that you may tolerate during exercise include bananas, energy bars, and fig newtons. Experiment to determine your own preferences and tolerances.

Experiment with various sports drinks to determine your favorite flavor and best tolerance. Consuming a variety of flavors may minimize the occurrence of taste fatigue during long exercise sessions and competitions. You may find that different products appeal to you in various athletic conditions. In hot and humid weather you may favor a product with little or no flavor. Know what works for you under various exercise, temperature, and race conditions.

Pay attention to signs of dehydration. Frequent gastrointestinal problems may indicate that you are not drinking enough. Gastric emptying is delayed when you are dehydrated. It may appear that you do not tolerate a particular product, when what is actually occurring is that the product is unable to empty from your stomach and subsequent drinking causes distention.

Pay attention to the signs and symptoms of hypoglycemia. Feeling light-headed, an inability to focus, and dizziness can all indicate that blood glucose levels are running low. Be proactive and try to increase your intake of carbohydrates with sports drinks, gels, or glucose tablets.

Keep fluid accessible during training and competition. Prepare bottles of sports drinks ahead of time. Pack your favorite gels and energy bars—learn to carry products. During long training sessions, packets of powdered sports drinks can be reconstituted with water so that you don't run out of fuel.

Refine your drinking technique. Practice drinking in all types of training situations. Know your limits regarding exercise intensity and the ability to tolerate certain volumes of fluid ingestion. Push your limits and maximize your fluid intake.

Pay attention to your sodium intake during ultraendurance events. Several days prior to competition emphasize salty foods and add salt to foods to taste. Choose higher sodium sports drinks, and add 1/8–1/4 teaspoon of sodium to each bottle of fluid if needed. Athletes who have difficulty maintaining sodium levels can take low dose sodium tablets with plenty of fluid.

Practice using liquid meal replacements or more concentrated drinks for consumption during ultraendurance events. These products are well tolerated by many ultraendurance athletes. They are low in fiber and bulk and empty from the stomach quickly. The small amounts of protein and fat they provide may also prevent hunger. Experiment with these products in training.

Avoid drinks high in fructose. Products that provide only fructose, a high concentration of fructose, or high fructose corn syrup may cause gastrointestinal upset.

Table 5.5 provides guidelines for using several types of sports nutrition products. Appendix C provides a comparison chart of sports drinks and liquid food supplements. When you consume a wide variety of sports nutrition supplements over the course of a day, or even a week, it is important to consider the other nutrients they provide such as vitamins and minerals. Consider your intake in the context of your entire day's food intake and be careful not to oversupplement on vitamins and minerals through use of these

5.5

PRACTICAL USES FOR SPORTS NUTRITION PRODUCTS

Sports Drinks
- Consume 16–24 ounces in the hour before exercise
- Consume 4– 8 ounces every 15–20 minutes during exercise
- Consume after exercise with a more concentrated carbohydrate source

Sports Gel
- Consume 1 packet in the hour prior to racing
- Consume 1 packet with 20 ounces of fluid during exercise when well hydrated
- Consume as part of recovery nutrition plan supplying total of 50–100 grams carbohydrates

Sports Bar
- Consume as part of pre-exercise meal
- Consume in the hour before racing if tolerated
- Consume during ultraendurance event if solid food is required and tolerated
- Consume as part of your immediate post-exercise recovery nutrition plan

High Carbohydrate Energy Drink
- Consume 16–32 ounces in the 1–2 hours prior to exercise
- May be consumed during an ultraendurance event if tolerated
- Consume for post-exercise carbohydrate

chapter 6

CREATING THE OPTIMAL TRAINING DIET

Meal Planning for Athletes

YOUR DAILY MEAL PLAN

As an endurance athlete who strives for optimal training and recovery, it is essential to translate sound scientific recommendations into everyday food choices that replenish your body fuel stores and leave you feeling satisfied with your diet. Much of the success of your daily eating plan will hinge on consuming adequate calories and carbohydrates that match your training program for that day (and the next day) and rounding out your meals and snacks with the correct balance of healthy proteins and fats.

Meal planning is not as complicated as it may sound. In fact, you will be amazed at how quickly you can adopt some new food strategies and incorporate them into your daily life of training and eating once you have a program and some structure in place. You will find that planning and organization makes this part of your training program easier and more effective. Just as you plan ahead to ensure that all the necessary equipment and clothing is available for your training plan, you must also plan to ensure that the optimal foods and required sports nutrition supplements are available to support your training. Table 6.1 summarizes the range of nutritional requirements for calories, carbohydrates, proteins, and fats for

NUTRITIONAL REQUIREMENTS OF ENDURANCE ATHLETES BASED ON TRAINING LEVELS

CALORIES (calories/lb. weight)	CARBOHYDRATES (g/lb. weight)	PROTEINS (g/lb. weight)	FATS (g/lb. weight)
Mild: 12–14 **Moderate:** 15–17 **High:** 18–24 **Very high:** 24–29	**Mild/Moderate:** 2.25–3.0 **Moderate/High:** 3.0–4.5 **High/Very High:** 4.5–5.5	**Moderate:** 0.45 **High:** 0.5–0.75 **Very High:** 0.8–0.9	> 0.5 depending on energy needs
160-lb. athlete with high activity level: 2,800–3,800 calories	560 g carbohydrate (60% calories)	128 g protein (13% calories)	115 g fat (27% calories)

endurance athletes. This table also outlines the total calorie, carbohydrate, protein, and fat requirements of a 160-pound athlete.

How these recommended nutrient amounts are translated into specific food choices and serving sizes can initially be one of the most difficult aspects of adopting the performance diet that best supports your training and sport. In real life, an individualized plan can differ from athlete to athlete depending on medical history, food preferences, schedule, and culinary skills. But food charts can be helpful in making carbohydrate servings more accessible.

Carbohydrates are often the central theme of your diet for several reasons:

- Running low on liver and muscle glycogen can impair your endurance training efforts long before depletion of other body fuels slows you down.
- Your carbohydrate intake is directly linked to the amount of glycogen you store in your liver and muscles, and these stores are relatively limited even with the proper diet.
- On certain training days you require a large amount of carbohydrates to replenish your muscle glycogen stores, and if you don't consume these amounts, your

muscle glycogen stores may not be adequate to properly fuel your subsequent training efforts.

■ Consuming these carbohydrate amounts takes planning, as the amounts you require often exceed what is found in an everyday diet, and if you leave your diet to chance your intake may be inadequate.

Food tables providing 10- to 30-gram carbohydrate portions can make meal planning smoother for the endurance athlete. You receive carbohydrates from several food groups: the bread, cereal, and grain group; the fruit and fruit juice group; the vegetable group; and the milk and yogurt group. You can match up the number of servings you require from these carbohydrate-containing groups to meet your requirements for training and recovery. On days when your carbohydrate needs are especially high, grains and starches are likely to comprise a good portion of your diet. They are concentrated food sources and provide 30 grams of carbohydrate per serving. As discussed in Chapter 2, try to choose lightly processed or whole grain sources as much as possible. Many items from the grain group such as pretzels and crackers also make good snack choices.

Fruits, dried fruit, and fruit juices, which also provide 30 grams per serving, are your next great source of carbohydrates and are excellent food choices for maintaining good health due to the abundant nutrients they supply. Vegetables are also sources of carbohydrates though not as high per portion as grains and fruits at 10 grams per serving. However, few foods can match vegetables for their high nutrient content.

Dairy milk, yogurt, soy milk, and rice milk are also good sources of carbohydrates ranging anywhere from 12 to 50 grams per serving. Yogurts can be especially high in carbohydrates when they come mixed with fruit and sugars. One last source of concentrated carbohydrates is sweets and desserts, which also supply 30 grams per serving. Sweets should not routinely replace more wholesome carbohydrate choices in your diet, but they are a great source of additional carbohydrates. They offer the advantage of being dense and less filling than some higher fiber, more wholesome choices, and when your carbohydrate requirements are especially high (exceeding 500 grams daily) these foods are handy choices. For very heavy training days, you can also consider adding some sports nutrition products high in carbohydrate to your food plan.

But of course endurance athletes cannot live and should not live on carbohydrates alone. Choosing quality proteins and healthy fats will provide you with essential nutrients and balance out your meals and snacks. Proteins and fats also keep you full longer and even out blood glucose levels during the day. Protein foods are ranked according to their fat content so that you do not exceed healthy limits of total fat and saturated fat in your diet. Plant proteins and milk and dairy sources are also emphasized for vegetarian athletes. Fats are also organized according to the types of fat they provide, so that you can choose healthy essential fatty acids and foods high in monounsaturated fat.

Table 6.2 outlines some of the serving recommendations for various calorie levels. This table is intended to be a framework from which you can base your own individual food choices. You may find that you prefer to do a bit of shuffling with the suggested food groups and number of servings to suit your own health goals and personal tastes. For example, some of the suggested daily plans may be too high in dairy foods for your own tastes. These plans can be modified and the carbohydrate intake maintained by adding the equivalent grams of carbohydrate servings from fruits and juices, or perhaps substituting soy milk for dairy milk. You may also wish to have fewer grain servings and increase the number of servings from fruits and fruit juices to match your carbohydrate requirements on certain training days. However, regardless of your personalized food plan and preferences, you need to reach the recommended carbohydrate amounts for optimal recovery and can add up the carbohydrates in the manner that best suits you. Of course, the nutrition guidelines presented in Chapter 2 should also direct you in making quality food choices as often as possible.

One useful tool for helping to determine if you are meeting your energy and nutrient requirements is a food journal. You are quite possibly already familiar with keeping

6.2

SERVING RECOMMENDATIONS FOR VARIOUS CALORIE LEVELS

Food Groups	CALORIE LEVELS				
	2,000	2,400	2,900	3,400	4,000
Grains	6	7	8	10	12
Fruits	3	3	4	5	6
Vegetables	2	3	3	3	3
Milk/Soy milk/ Yogurt	2	2	2 (milk) 1 (yogurt)	2 (milk) 1 (yogurt)	3 (milk) 1 (yogurt)
Protein	6	6	6	7	8
Fats	3	4	5	6	8
Carbohydrate	315 g	350 g	450 g	550 g	650 g
Protein	84 g	112 g	114 g	120 g	150 g
Fat	45 g	60 g	70 g	80 g	89 g

a training journal and have learned what a good tool it is for fine-tuning your training program. To reap the most benefits from keeping a food journal, it is best if you write down your food choices and portions while eating or immediately after eating. Don't forget to mark snacks, supplements, and any fluids consumed. With help from the food lists provided, you can assess a number of items regarding your food intake:

- Add up the amount of carbohydrate grams you consume in one day and determine if your intake matches your training efforts. Note not only if your daily totals are adequate, but also if the amount of carbohydrates you consume before and after exercise is appropriate to support your training and recovery efforts.
- Record the amount of fluids and carbohydrates that you consume during exercise. Determine if you meet the recommended fluid amounts and intake up to 0.5 grams per pound of weight or 30–75 grams per hour.
- Look through the day's intake to ensure that adequate sources of concentrated and high quality proteins are being consumed. If you are a vegetarian, check that your portions of plant proteins are full portions so that your body receives all the required amino acids.

- Determine if the fats you consume are derived from healthy monounsaturated and polyunsaturated food choices. Check that you consume good sources of essential fatty acids in your diet.
- Measure your intake of hydrating fluids for the day, and before and after training. Make sure that you are hyperhydrated before exercise and that you consume enough fluid to replace sweat losses after exercise.
- Check for hidden fats such as those found in muffins, pastries, and high fat crackers. Try to minimize your intake of these foods whenever possible.
- Pay attention to your eating patterns. Note if there are times during the day when you become too hungry and adjust your mealtimes accordingly. Pay attention to any eating that may occur due to boredom, stress, and other issues not related to hunger.

Tables 6.3, 6.4, and 6.5 are provided for sports nutrition meal planning. These lists provide serving and carbohydrate amounts for the major foods that can comprise a well-balanced sports nutrition diet. The protein foods are ranked according to fat content so that you may select the leanest choices available and limit your intake of saturated fat. The fats are also grouped according to types of fat so that you may make the healthiest choices possible.

PLANNING YOUR DAILY MEALS

Meal planning does not need to be a frustrating experience for dedicated endurance athletes. It isn't necessary to employ your own personal chef for quick gourmet meals. But like your training program, meal planning does require forethought, organization, and flexibility. With practice, your meal planning skills will become second nature. Some of the fundamentals of meal planning follow.

Have a well-organized and well-equipped kitchen. Make sure that you have all the convenience items that you need including a microwave, steamer, toaster oven, microwave-proof cookware, and a slow cooker. Other handy items include

6.3

CARBOHYDRATE CONTENT OF FOODS

30 G CARBOHYDRATE SERVINGS FOR CEREALS, STARCHES, GRAINS

Breads

Bagel	1/2 large or 2 oz.
Bread	2 slices or 2 oz.
Bread crumbs	1/2 cup
Bread sticks	2 oz.
Cornbread	1 square or 2 oz.
Dinner rolls	2 oz.
English muffin	1 whole or 2 oz.
Hamburger bun	1 whole or 2 oz.
Pita pocket	1 round or 2 oz.

Cereals

Bran cereal	2/3 cup
Cereal, cold, unsweetened	1.5 oz.
Cream of wheat, cooked	1 cup
Granola, low fat	1/2 cup
Grape-Nuts	1/3 cup or 5 Tbsp.
Grits, cooked	1 cup
Oatmeal, cooked	1 cup
Puffed cereal	3 cups
Shredded wheat	3/4 cup or 1.5 oz.

Grains

Barley, raw	1/4 cup
Buckwheat, raw	1/4 cup
Bulgar, cooked	3/4 cup
Crackers	1.5 oz.
Muffin, low fat	3 oz.
Pancakes	3, 4-inch diameter
Pancake mix, dry	1/3 cup
Pasta, cooked	1 cup
Pretzels	1.5 oz.
Rice, cooked	2/3 cup
Rice milk	1 cup
Saltines	8 crackers or 1.5 oz.
Tortilla, corn or flour	2

Starchy Vegetables

Baked beans, cooked	3/4 cup
Corn, cooked	3/4 cup
Kidney beans, cooked	3/4 cup
Peas, cooked	1 cup
Potato, baked	1 medium or 5 oz.
Sweet potato, baked	4 oz.

Table 6.3 continued on next page

CARBOHYDRATE CONTENT OF FOODS *continued*

30 G CARBOHYDRATE SERVINGS—FRUIT

Apple	1 1/2 medium
Apples, dried	7 rings
Applesauce, sweetened	1/2 cup
Applesauce, unsweetened	1 cup
Apricots, fresh	8 medium
Banana	1 large
Blueberries	1 1/2 cups
Cantaloupe, raw pieces	2 cups
Dates, dried	1 fruit
Figs, dried	3 whole
Fruit salad	1 cup
Grapefruit	1 large
Grapes	30 or 1 cup
Kiwifruit	3 medium
Mango	1 medium
Nectarine	2 small
Orange	2 medium
Papaya	1 whole
Peach	2 medium
Pear	1 large
Pineapple, fresh, pieces	1 1/2 cups
Plum	3 medium
Raisins	1/3 cup or 3 Tbsp.
Raspberries	2 cups
Strawberries	2.5 cups
Watermelon	3 slices or 3 cups

30 G CARBOHYDRATE SERVINGS—FRUIT AND VEGETABLE JUICES

Apple juice	8 oz.
Carrot juice	10 oz.
Cranberry juice cocktail	8 oz.
Grape juice	8 oz.
Grapefruit juice	8 oz.
Orange juice	8 oz.
Pineapple juice	8 oz.
Vegetable juice cocktail	24 oz.

CARBOHYDRATE CONTENT OF FOODS *continued*

10 G CARBOHYDRATE SERVINGS—VEGETABLES

Artichoke	1 medium
Asparagus, boiled	1 cup
Beans, green, boiled	1 cup
Beet greens, cooked	1 1/4 cups
Broccoli, boiled	1 cup
Broccoli, raw	2 cups
Brussels sprouts, boiled	3/4 cup
Cabbage, cooked	3/4 cup
Carrots, cooked	2/3 cup
Carrots, raw	2 medium
Cauliflower, cooked	3/4 cup
Kale, boiled	1 1/4 cups
Mushrooms, cooked	1 cup
Mustard greens, cooked	1 1/2 cups
Peppers, sweet, raw	2 cups
Spinach, boiled	1 1/2 cups
Summer squash, cooked	1 cup
Tomato, raw 1 medium	2

12–50 G CARBOHYDRATE SERVINGS—MILK AND YOGURT

Milk, 1%	8 oz. (12 g)	Yogurt, low fat	8 oz. (15 to 20 g)
Milk, 2%	8 oz. (12 g)	Yogurt, nonfat	8 oz. (15 g)
Milk, buttermilk, 1%	8 oz. (12 g)	Yogurt, soy	8 oz. (30 g)
Milk, nonfat	8 oz. (12 g)	Yogurt, with fruit	8 oz. (30 to 45 g)
Milk, rice	8 oz. (28 g)		
Milk, soy	8 oz. (22 g)		

30 G CARBOHYDRATE SERVINGS—SWEET AND BAKED GOODS

Angel food cake	1/12 whole	Jam or jelly	2 Tbsp.
Cake	1/12 whole	Pie	1/8 whole
Chocolate milk	8 oz.	Pudding, regular	1/2 cup
Cookie, fat free	4 small	Sherbet	1/2 cup
Fruit spreads, 100% fruit	2 Tbsp.	Sorbet	1/2 cup
Gingersnaps	6 cookies	Syrup, regular	2 Tbsp.
Graham crackers	6 squares	Vanilla wafers	10
Granola bar, low fat	1 bar	Yogurt, frozen, low fat	1 cup
Honey	2 Tbsp.	Yogurt, frozen, fat free	2/3 cup
Ice cream	1 cup		

PROTEIN CHOICES GROUPED ACCORDING TO FAT CONTENT

	FAT PROTEIN			
Very low (< 2 g fat/oz.)	Low (3–4 g fat/oz.)	Medium (4–5 g fat/oz.)	High (6–8 g fat/oz.)	Very high (> 8 g fat/oz.)
FISH Shellfish: Clams Crab Lobster Shrimp White fish: Bass Grouper Haddock Halibut Sole Tuna	Dark fish: Mackerel Salmon Sardines	Salmon and tuna packed in oil		Any fried fish product
CHEESE Cottage cheese, 1% Cottage cheese, 2% Fat free cheese	Low fat cheeses	Feta cheese Mozzarella, part-skim Parmesan, grated	Mozzarella Neufchatel	American, processed Brie Cheddar Cream cheese Edam Limburger Monterey Muenster Swiss
BEEF Round, choice, 90% lean	Flank steak, choice Porterhouse, choice Rib-eye, choice Round, choice, 85% lean	Round, choice, 73% lean Round, choice, 80% lean	Roast beef Meatloaf	Corned beef Prime cuts Short ribs

6.4

PROTEIN CHOICES GROUPED ACCORDING TO FAT CONTENT

FAT PROTEIN

Very low (< 2 g fat/oz.)	Low (3–4 g fat/oz.)	Medium (4–5 g fat/oz.)	High (6–8 g fat/oz.)	Very high (> 8 g fat/oz.)
PORK Boneless sirloin Chop Ham, lean, 95% fat free Pork tenderloin Top loin chop	Blade steak Boneless rib roast Canadian bacon Center loin chop Center rib chop Sirloin roast	Pork butt	Italian sausage	Bacon Pastrami Pate Pork Sausage
LAMB Leg, top round Leg, shank, half	Loin chop Loin roast Rib chop	Roast lamb		Ground lamb
LEGUMES (per cup) Black beans Kidney beans Lentils Lima beans Pinto beans		Chickpeas	Tofu	Soybeans
POULTRY Chicken, white, no skin Turkey breast Turkey, dark, no Skin	Chicken, dark, no skin Chicken, dark, w/skin Duck, roasted, no skin Turkey, dark, w/skin	Ground turkey, mixed meat/skin	Duck, roasted, w/skin	
OTHER Egg substitute Egg whites Luncheon meat, 95% fat-free	Egg Substitute Luncheon meat, 86% fat free	Eggs	Bologna Hotdogs Luncheon meat Turkey/chicken	Beef/pork hotdogs Bratwurst Knockwurst Peanut butter Salami

a large stovetop skillet or wok, a rice cooker, a lasagna dish, and sharp knives. Knowing where all your items are located and feeling comfortable in your kitchen will make putting together quick and easy meals that much easier.

Plan out your week's meal ideas beforehand. Think ahead to what meals you will need to cook, pack, or eat out based on that week's schedule. Determine how many dinners you will cook that week and leave room for healthy takeout, eating out, and leftovers. Think about where you will be for lunch. Do you need to pack a full lunch or some extras like pretzels and fruit? Determine if your training schedule requires you to have energy bars or carbohydrate drinks on hand. Perhaps you prefer quick recovery nutrition items to tide you over until your next full meal. You may want to be very specific and have certain days of the week designated for specific types of meals. For example, Monday night could be chicken, while Thursday is fish and Friday is stir-fry. Try to vary the types of vegetables and sides you consume. Sometimes it is easier to obtain variety when dinner is prepared for an entire family. When cooking for just one to two persons, try to obtain variety on a weekly basis, switching the grains, fruits, and vegetables you consume.

6.5

SOURCES OF FAT

Polyunsaturated fat (5 g serving)	Monounsaturated fat (5 g serving)	Saturated fat (5 g serving)
Margarine, stick, tub, or squeeze, 1 tsp. lower-fat, 1 Tbsp.	Avocado, medium, 1/8	Butter, stick, 1 tsp. reduced fat, 1 Tbsp. whipped, 1 tsp.
Mayonnaise, regular, 1 tsp. reduced fat, 1 Tbsp.	Bacon, cooked, 1 slice Nuts:	Cream, half-and-half, 2 Tbsp.
Nuts, walnuts, 4 halves	Almonds, cashews, 6 nuts	Shortening or lard, 1 tsp.
Oil, corn, safflower, soy-bean, flaxseed, walnut, 1 tsp.	Peanuts, 10 nuts Pecans, 4 halves	Sour cream, regular, 2 Tbsp.
Pumpkin seeds, 1 Tbsp.	Oil, Canola, olive, peanut, 1 tsp.	reduced fat, 3 Tbsp.
Salad Dressing, regular, 1 Tbsp.	Olives, black, 8 large	
Sunflower seeds, 1 Tbsp.	Peanut butter, 2 tsp.	
	Sesame seeds, 1 Tbsp.	
	Tahini paste, 2 tsp.	

Keep non-perishable stock food items amply supplied. Having a well-stocked cupboard of items like rice, pasta, whole grains, instant couscous, and other dry items can save you in a pinch when fresh food supplies run low or during heavy training weeks. Some quick meals made from these ingredients include black bean burritos (freeze the tortillas), pasta and tomato sauce, stir-fry made from frozen chicken, instant rice, frozen vegetable mixes, and canned chili with bread or crackers. A suggested stock list is provided in Table 6.6.

Go grocery shopping every week for fresh items. Have a designated grocery shopping day and time and make it part of your weekly schedule. Based on your food plan for the week, put together a shopping list. Don't wait to shop when it is convenient, as it may never be convenient! You also don't want to set yourself up for several quick trips to the store to grab a few needed items. In the long run, this will cost you more time. Try to find a supermarket that can supply all the items you need. You will know where all your regular items are located and save time. Go during off-peak times to avoid crowds and don't mull over items that are not on your shopping list. If you can't make it to the supermarket some weeks, try an increasingly popular alternative and find a grocery store or online grocery system that accepts phone, fax, or Internet orders and that delivers.

Keep a running list of items that need to be replenished. Have a pad and pen handy. When you notice that items are running low or are used up, add them to your list. Trying to remember everything you need while shopping at the grocery store may not be the best strategy for a busy athlete.

Batch cook meals, make extra portions, and freeze single servings. This strategy can be a great time saver. You can set aside a lighter training day to cook items such as soup, chili, and lasagna. When cooking regular meals, making an extra one to two portions for the next day can save dinner preparation time or provide you with a nice midday meal. Freeze single item portions in plastic containers for future heavy training days.

Pack meals, snacks, and food supplements for the next training day the night before. If your next day's schedule is full, consider packing your foods and snacks the

6.6

SIMPLE SUGGESTIONS FOR STOCKING YOUR PANTRY

FOR THE FREEZER

Chicken tenders	Textured vegetable proteins	Frozen vegetables
Cooked shrimp	Variety of breads	Stir-fry mixes
Lean ground beef	Waffles	Sorbet
Lean pork filets	English muffins	Frozen fruit
Cubed meat for stir-fry	Muffins	Pre-cooked pasta and rice
Soy and garden burgers	Tortillas	Egg substitute

FOR THE REFRIGERATOR

Fresh fruit	Reduced fat cheese	Soy and rice milk
Fresh vegetables	Pre-washed salad greens	Sauces and condiments
Juices	Mini carrots	Salsa
Milk	Oranges, apples, bananas	Tub margarine
Yogurt	Lean deli meats	
Eggs	Fresh pasta	

FOR THE CUPBOARD

Pasta	Canned Tuna	Granola bars
Rice	Peanut butter	Canned soup
Couscous	Instant stuffing mixes	Nuts and sunflower seeds
Quinoa	Low fat crackers	Pretzels
Pilaf	Cold cereal assortment	Instant soup and grain
Tabouleh	Oatmeal and farina	cups
Canned beans and	Dried fruit	Fig newtons
chickpeas		Seasoning mixes

night before. Having some portioned items and fresh food in the fridge will make this task as simple as possible. Plan snacks that can be eaten on the run.

Acquire a repertoire of quick and easy to prepare meals. Anyone can become a proficient cook, and it does not have to be a time-consuming project. Be on the lookout for quick and simple recipes. Ask friends for some of their quick meal ideas. Focus on recipes like stir-fry, risotto, burritos, and pastas.

Take advantage of food shortcuts. Purchase chicken tender strips, beef stir-fry strips, frozen pre-cooked shrimp, and rotisserie chickens. Try frozen vegetable stir-fry mixes, pre-cut fruits, pre-seasoned and cut tofu, ready to heat soups, instant couscous mixes, fresh pastas (you can freeze them), and canned beans, chickpeas, and other legumes.

Breakfast, Lunch, and Snacks

Breakfast is one of the most important meals of the day. It revs up your body's metabolism and refills liver glycogen stores that have become depleted overnight. It may even be an important recovery meal after a solid early morning training session. By skipping breakfast, eating a medium-size lunch, and feasting at dinner, you may not only be compromising your recovery but also cheating your body of important nutrients. Skipping breakfast is also a terrible weight management strategy that can set you up for increased hunger and overeating later in the day.

Breakfast will keep your digestive juices flowing, but may keep you feeling satisfied for only three hours or so until you are hungry again. If this occurs, insert a mid-morning snack into your eating plan. If your energy needs are high, try to have a substantial breakfast. Eat calorically dense cereals such as granola and muesli. A large glass of juice will also add a substantial amount of calories and carbohydrates. Adding some protein to your breakfast can help keep you comfortably full until the next meal. Depending on your schedule, you may consume breakfast on the fly. Quick choices can include a fruit smoothie made with yogurt and granola. Quick-packs include yogurt, bananas, dried fruit, bagels, and muffins. Table 6.7 lists some breakfast ideas.

For many athletes, lunch will either be brought from home or purchased at a restaurant or fast-food establishment. Like all your meals and snacks, lunch should provide some quality carbohydrates and be balanced out with protein and fat. Eat lunch when hunger first sets in, as this is a sign that your body needs fuel.

Packing a lunch takes a little extra time and planning but is well worth the effort. You can ensure that you have lean proteins and the right type and amount of fats. Sandwiches are always a good place to start when last night's leftovers seem too repetitive. Some good protein options are lean beef, hummus, turkey, chicken, tuna, and low fat cottage cheese. Liven up that turkey sandwich with add-ons such as avocado, lettuce leaves, cucumber, tomato, sprouts, and low fat cheese. High carbohydrate items that you can include with your lunch are fruits, pretzels, raw vegetables, yogurt, low fat chips, low fat crackers, and vegetable and bean soups.

Snacks are also a very important part of an endurance athlete's diet. When your energy needs are high, snacks give you a nice calorie boost. They also provide some fuel before training sessions and keep hunger at bay until you can sit down for a full meal. Many elite athletes swear by snacking. Plan some serious snacking into your diet. If there is a particular time of day when you experience an energy low or hunger, snacking may make all the difference. Table 6.8 lists some tasty snack ideas.

6.7
BREAKFAST IDEAS
Cooked oatmeal with raisins, cinnamon, and low fat milk
Open-face English muffin halves with broiled cheese and fruit
Egg substitute omelet with vegetables, toast, juice, and milk
Yogurt with fresh fruit and a low fat muffin
Whole grain cereal with milk and fruit
Fruit smoothie made with yogurt, fresh or frozen fruit, and granola
Whole grain bread with peanut butter, banana, and honey
Any leftovers that sound appealing

LABEL READING TIPS

Nutritional information on labels can help you determine the nutritional breakdown of foods. First check the ingredient list. You may want to include more whole wheat flours and other whole grains into your diet. Ingredients are listed in the labels by weight from the most to the least.

Pay attention to the serving size on the label and compare it to the amount that you actually eat. The portions you consume may be double those on the package, and you should adjust the nutrition information accordingly. You can also use the label to evaluate if a food will significantly impact your carbohydrate intake by checking the total grams of carbohydrates listed. You can then determine what portion of that particular food would provide 30 or more grams of carbohydrates to help you meet your training requirements.

6.8

SMART SNACKS TO KEEP YOUR TANK TOPPED OFF

Cereal, with or without milk

Peanut butter and jelly sandwich

Hard and soft pretzels

Baked potato with low fat cheese

Crackers with peanut butter

Muffins and bagels with jam and low fat cream cheese

Sports bars, breakfast bars, low fat granola bars

Yogurt with fruit

Bowl of soup with crackers

Pasta or bean salad

Fresh fruit, low fat cheese, and nuts

Cottage cheese and fruit

Instant breakfast mix and fruit

Tuna salad and crackers

Hummus and crackers or pita bread

Fruit smoothie

Milk chug and fruit

Total fat grams as well as calories from fat are also listed. To determine the percent calories from fat, divide the fat calories per serving by the total calories per serving and multiply by 100. Keep higher fat foods in perspective. Your fat intake needs to be considered in the context of an entire day. Your total day's intake should provide 20 to 25 percent fat calories, which allows for some healthy foods that may be a bit higher in fat. Some foods such as dried pasta will be very low in fat, while others such as margarine provide a high amount of fat.

The Daily Value for various vitamins and minerals provided on the nutrition label are based on a 2,000-calorie intake. The percent daily value can tell you if a food is high or low in a nutrient such as calcium, fiber, iron, or vitamin C. A food is considered to be a good source of a nutrient if it provides 20 percent of the Daily Value. Besides increasing your intake of foods high in specific nutrients, you can also use the Daily Value to avoid excess fat, saturated fat, and cholesterol.

DIETARY RULES FOR RESTAURANTS

Like many North Americans, chances are that you eat out several times weekly. Lunch is the meal most frequently eaten away from home, followed by dinner and then breakfast. Currently, more than 45 percent of money spent on food in the

United States goes to restaurant meals and other foods consumed away from home. You may eat out at restaurants, in a cafeteria, at your desk, and even in your car.

Regardless of where you eat your meal out, the basic strategies are the same. Watch out for hidden and added fat, and keep a close eye on the portions. Despite your high energy requirements for endurance training, not all restaurant meals fit nicely into your nutrition plan. They may be too high in fat to become a frequent indulgence and may not provide the healthy ingredients that you require. It is important to learn what healthy food choices are available at your favorite restaurants. Ask questions about how foods are prepared and don't hesitate to request modifications or changes. Often you can creatively outsmart the menu and enjoy your meal as well.

Fast-food

Fast-food can provide excessive amounts of protein and fat through supersize burgers and grease-laden French fries. But it is possible to make choices that fit into a sports diet at some fast-food establishments. Have the small hamburgers that provide only 2 or 3 ounces of meat. Order baked potatoes over French fries whenever possible. Broiled chicken sandwiches are decent choices, while chicken pieces are generally fried. The same goes for fish sandwiches, as they come dripping with plenty of unwanted oil. Order skim milk when possible. Juice is often available as well. Salads and vegetables may be on the menu, but watch out for dressings. Limit sauces and toppings whenever possible.

Many fast-food establishments now provide good sandwich choices. You can choose lean roast beef, ham, turkey, or chicken, and limit oils, mayonnaise, and cheese. Go for baked chips and pretzels when offered. Chicken fajitas or tacos make some good lower fat choices. You can also choose frozen yogurt and low fat milkshakes.

Other fast-food choices that can fit into your sports nutrition plan include vegetarian thin-crust pizza. Some establishments also have a soup and baked potato bar. Bean burritos and soft tacos are also available, as are chili, bagels, English muffins, waffles, pancakes, and cereals.

Ethnic Cuisine

Chances are if you eat out frequently that you enjoy many types of ethnic cuisine. These cultural edibles can fit into a healthy training diet if you know what choices to make and avoid consuming hidden fat.

Italian Cuisine

Italian food is a popular favorite and can be consumed at a variety of settings—upscale, family style, pizza, or fast-food. With an emphasis on grains and vegetables, Italian eating can be healthy. Some lighter, lower fat choices would be: starches such as spaghetti, risotto and polenta (prepared low fat), vegetable choices such as tomato based sauces, zucchini and other vegetables prepared without fat, and lean meats such as skinless chicken, veal, shrimp, and grilled fish. You can also try condiments like herbs, cooking wines, vinegar, garlic, and crushed red peppers. Fill up on minestrone soup, and top pasta with marinara or red clam sauce. Order your dressing on the side and have Italian ice for dessert. You can also make special requests, including removing the olive oil from the table and having the skin taken off chicken.

There are also plenty of heavier choices at Italian restaurants. Starches such as garlic bread and focaccia contain fat, as do fried vegetables and meats such as salami, prosciutto, and sausage. Watch out for high fat cheeses and dishes prepared with cream, butter, and even olive oil, which still contains plenty of fat calories. Go easy on the antipasto plate and the olive oil served with bread. Alfredo sauce, Italian sausage, lasagna, and parmigiana dishes are all high in fat because of the ingredients and methods of preparation.

Mexican Cuisine

Mexican cuisine may also be on your list of ethnic favorites. Like Italian food, this cuisine contains both light and heavy choices. Many staples of Mexican cuisine can be considered low fat items such as whole beans, refried beans prepared without

Protein and the Vegetarian Athlete

Endurance athletes do have increased protein requirements, and vegetarian athletes should appreciate that a portion of a quality plant protein is not as concentrated a source of protein as an animal protein. The key to obtaining enough protein in your diet is to first consume enough calories so that the protein you do consume is not processed for energy. Secondly, an emphasis must be placed upon high quality and concentrated plant protein sources. Certain grains, dried peas and beans, lentils, nuts, and seeds are some of the best sources. Soy products such as tempeh and tofu are one plant protein essentially equivalent to animal protein. While it is not necessary to combine or complement various plant proteins at the same meal as was once thought, you should make a concerted effort to obtain adequate plant proteins in your diet throughout the day. The body will make its own complete proteins over the course of the day if you consume enough calories. If your calorie intake falls short, some of the protein you do consume may be processed for energy rather than utilized for important protein functions. Table 6.9 lists some good plant protein sources.

Protein Tips for Vegetarians

- Include a protein rich food at all meals and snacks.
- Add milk or fortified soy milk or the yogurt equivalent to every meal or snack.
- Use nuts, butters, hummus, and low fat cheeses (soy and regular) for toppings on breads, bagels, and crackers.
- Add nuts and seeds to a fruit and yogurt snack.
- Make tofu and tempeh stir-fry.
- Experiment with quick and easy bean recipes such as burritos, casseroles, and salads.

- Make thick soups and stews with beans and lentils.
- Experiment with all the meat replacer soy products on the market such as tofu dogs and burgers.
- Make casseroles, lasagna, and stuffed shell recipes with tofu.

Meal Planning Tips for Vegetarians

- The health food sections of many supermarkets and most health food stores provide a wide selection of vegetarian food choices and convenience items.

(continued on page 140)

6.9

PLANT SOURCES OF PROTEIN

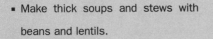

Food	Portion	Protein (grams)
Tempeh	1 cup	39.0
Soybeans, cooked	1 cup	29.0
Seitan	4 oz.	21.0
Tofu, firm	4 oz.	20.0
Lentils, cooked	1 cup	18.0
Black beans, cooked	1 cup	15.0
Chickpeas, cooked	1 cup	15.0
Kidney beans, cooked	1 cup	15.0
Lima beans, cooked	1 cup	15.0
Pinto beans, cooked	1 cup	14.0
Quinoa, cooked	1 cup	11.0
Soy milk	1 cup	10.0
Soy yogurt	1 cup	10.0
Tofu, regular	4 oz.	10.0
Peanut butter	2 Tbsp.	8.0
Peas, cooked	1 cup	8.0
Sunflower seeds	1/4 cup	8.0
Bagel	1 medium	6.0
Bulgar, cooked	1 cup	6.0
Pasta or grain	1 cup cooked	6.0
Almonds	1/4 cup	5.5
Bread, whole wheat	2 slices	5.0
Brown rice, cooked	1 cup	5.0
Potato	1 medium	4.5

(continued from page 139)

- The number of textured vegetable protein products has increased significantly in the past several years. You can now buy products that resemble and taste like hotdogs, burgers, and breakfast sausage. Many of these products make quick and easy lunch ideas.

- Tofu can be substituted for chicken in most recipes. Seasoned tofu is available, and you can also season the recipe to spice up tofu's milder taste.

- You can substitute vegetable broth when recipes call for beef or chicken stock. Vegetable broth is available in many supermarkets and most health food stores.

- Canned lentils, chickpeas, and beans are a quick and nutritious vegetarian option. When time allows, soak the dried lentil and bean versions. Many bean and lentil recipes can be batch cooked and frozen for later use.

- If you need assistance, find a vegetarian cookbook that provides meal ideas suited to athletes.

- Include protein rich foods at each meal. Because vegetarian options are not as concentrated in protein as animal protein, you need to include adequate portions at most meals and snacks.

- Purchase calcium fortified soy and rice milks if you drink these products instead of dairy milk.

- Purchase iron fortified cereals and consume them with products high in vitamin C such as orange juice. ■

oil, tortillas, rice cooked without oil, grilled vegetables, and salsa. Grilled proteins such as shrimp, fish, or chicken are good choices, as are whole black beans. You can also fill up on gazpacho, marinated vegetables, and burritos (easy on the cheese).

Some heavier choices at Mexican restaurants would be tortilla chips, chimichangas, and taco shells. Avocados (guacamole), olives, sour cream, and cheese are also high in fat. You should also watch out for chorizo, cheese, sour cream, and oil used in cooking as they may contribute a significant amount of fat and saturated fat to your diet.

Chinese Cuisine

Finally, Chinese cuisine providing a variety of regional cooking styles is a frequent favorite at mall eateries and small neighborhood restaurants. While there are light choices in Chinese cooking, there are also many high fat pitfalls. To keep your meal on the light side, look for stir-fried vegetables. You have a variety to choose from like peapods, bamboo shoots, water chestnuts, cabbage, baby corn, and broccoli.

Lean proteins that are found in Chinese dishes include vegetable dishes with shrimp, chicken, tofu, and lean cuts of beef and pork. Dishes may also contain low fat fruits such as pineapple and orange sections. Condiments like mustard, soy sauce, ginger, sweet sauce, and garlic will not increase the fat content of your meals.

Chinese cuisine also contains plenty of high fat choices. Everyone is familiar with the fatty breaded and fried sweet and sour dishes. Fried rice has twice the calories as steamed rice, with all the additional calories coming from oil. Fried noodles and egg rolls can also up your fat intake. Try to stay away from fried seafood, pork, spare ribs, and duck with skin. Stir-fry dishes that contain nuts and peanuts will also be much higher in fat, as will any choices in which oil is used heavily. Request that your dish be prepared with as little oil as possible, and try to split entrees as portions are often large.

Salad Bars

Visits to the salad bar are often well intended but can result in surprisingly high fat meals. Beside those healthy raw vegetable items like spinach, tomatoes, broccoli, and green peppers are plenty of items mixed with fat or sitting in oil. Some of the less healthy choices include pasta salad, potato salad, marinated vegetables, cheeses, and bean salads made with oil. Go easy on portions of these items. Of course, try to keep salad dressing portions reasonable.

Salad bars have plenty of carbohydrates and fiber and can help you keep your protein portions low and reasonable. Obviously fresh greens and plain raw vegetables are your best choices. Starches on the salad bar may include chickpeas, kidney beans, green peas, crackers, and pita bread. Lean protein salad bar choices include plain tuna, cottage cheese, egg, ham, and feta cheese. Try to avoid most cheeses and pepperoni. Keep marinated vegetable portions small, and especially watch out for tuna, chicken, seafood salad, macaroni salad, and potato salads that can contain plenty of mayonnaise. High fat items including peanuts, sesame seeds, and sunflower seeds provide good fats and can be used in small amounts.

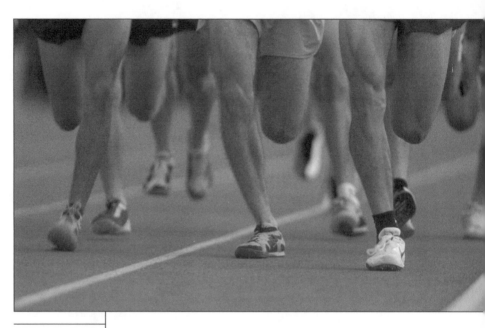

TOM MORAN PHOTO

chapter 7

WEIGHT AND CHANGING BODY COMPOSITION

Becoming Lean and Strong

Endurance athletes come in a variety of shapes and sizes, often demonstrating a physique and body composition suited to their sport. However, because of data on elite athletes correlating lower levels of body fat to improved performance, athletes often become overly focused on body weight and size. Frequently endurance athletes attempt to modify their body composition by decreasing levels of body fat and/or increasing levels of muscle mass.

There are smart and sensible ways to attain a lean and strong body. However, there are also many destructive ways to attain an overly idealized body composition that may not be realistic for your lifestyle, level of training, or genetics. It is easy to assume that dropping a few "extra" pounds will allow you to bike, run, ski, and swim faster, but athletic success is not always that simple. There are many examples of athletes at all levels who have restricted their diet in attempts to improve body composition, ultimately resulting in a decrease in energy levels and performance. It is important that you keep an open mind regarding your "best" weight. Don't compromise recovery and energy for a few pounds. There is no point in possessing a lean or thin body if you don't have the strength and energy to move that body up hills, over terrain, and through water at your desired race pace.

STEPPING ON THE SCALE

It is important that you keep the scale in perspective, as it provides only a rudimentary measure of your body weight. The scale weighs all of you—muscle, fat, bone, water, body organs—and does not differentiate between these body tissues. For this reason, highly muscular athletes may weigh at the high end of their "ideal" weight. Conversely, thin, small-boned people weigh less and are favored by the scale. Obviously your body weight is influenced by much more than what you eat and how much you train. Many of the factors that affect your weight are determined by genetics and are basically out of your control.

The best use of a weight scale is to monitor long-term changes over time as they coincide with monitored body composition changes, and to measure short-term changes related to your hydration status. As mentioned previously, weight loss after a hard training session provides feedback regarding your level of hydration. It is recommended that for every pound of weight lost during exercise, you rehydrate with 24 ounces of non-caffeinated fluid.

Long-term weight changes as measured by a scale can provide you with a crude indicator regarding changes in body composition over time or even help you determine if you are keeping up with your energy needs. Chronic unwanted weight loss can indicate that you are not meeting your caloric requirements and perhaps pushing yourself to an overtrained state. It is also important to not get overly focused on an idealized weight obtained from a height and weight chart or on the weight and body fat levels of a top competitor in your sport. While certain body fat averages have been measured for specific sports, there are a number of individual and interconnected factors other than body fat that affect an athlete's performance. Averages also indicate that athletes can be successful at varying degrees of reasonable body fat levels, with some competitors at the low end of the body fat range and others at the high end. Top athletes do not always fit the lean ideal for their sport, and a low body fat level does not guarantee success.

BODY FAT LEVELS

It is important to appreciate how your body fat levels reflect upon good health. Your total body fat consists of both essential fat and stored fat. Your brain, nervous system, and other body structures rely upon essential fat for proper functioning. Generally, though with some variation, males need to store at least 5 percent body fat for proper body functioning and females 12 percent. Storage fat, the fat that most endurance athletes do not want to carry on a long run or hilly bike ride, is simply excess stored energy. Storage fat surrounds your organs, but a substantial amount is located under the skin. Your performance could possibly improve with body fat loss, but only if you truly have unneeded fat to lose. Most men are healthy at 15 to 18 percent body fat and women at 20 to 25 percent body fat. Lean endurance athletes often fall at 5 to 10 percent body fat for men and 10 to 15 percent body fat for women.

Very low body fat levels can have a negative effect on both your health and performance. A thin athlete is not necessarily a strong athlete. Excess or rapid weight loss can compromise your immune system and result in muscle loss and decreased power output. Rather than choosing some arbitrary body fat level, it is important to determine a level that is best for you. Your ideal body fat level should:

- Not be based on the minimum levels.
- Not be based on that of a top competitor.
- Account for individuality and genetics.
- Be in accordance with good health.
- Not require extreme dieting or training to reach and maintain.

There are two valid reasons to check your body fat percentage. First, you can determine how changes in your diet and training affect your levels of body fat, and therefore muscle or lean body mass levels. Secondly, you can also determine what body fat levels are associated with your best performance and sense of well being.

Techniques for Measuring Body Fat Levels

Regardless of the body fat measurement technique that you employ, you should keep in mind that all techniques measure your body fat indirectly. When choosing a body fat measurement technique, you should consider the following guidelines:

- The technique and formula used to estimate your body fat should be valid for endurance athletes of your sex and age.
- A reliable technician should perform the technique.
- The same technique should be repeated over time to obtain long-term data and to measure progressive changes.
- The results should be interpreted by a knowledgeable expert who is aware of the limitations of the technique and can advise you appropriately.

The following body fat measurement techniques are most commonly utilized. They all contain some inherent error in their technique and provide only an estimate of body composition. No one method is absolutely accurate, and accuracy can vary among techniques. Clearly, the measurement of body composition is far from being an exact science. For example, a commonly utilized technique is skinfold testing, which has a standard error of 3 percent. If an athlete were to test at 15 percent body fat, actual body fat levels could range from 12 to 18 percent. Body fat assessments provide a possible range rather than an absolute number.

Hydrostatic Weighing

Hydrostatic or underwater weighing is a water displacement technique often cited as the "gold standard" of body fat assessment, despite having a standard error of at least 2 percent. Hydrostatic weighing involves being weighed under water after expelling all the air from your lungs. Your body density is then estimated from the difference between your weight on land and your weight under water. Your body fat is then extrapolated from this information.

Like all methods, hydrostatic weighing is not error free. This method assumes a constant fat free body density and may not be appropriate for all population groups. Underwater weighing can be a bit uncomfortable but is offered at some sports medicine centers and universities. Your health club may have someone perform this technique several times throughout the year.

Air Displacement

Also known as body plethysmography, this technique also measures body density, but by air displacement rather than water displacement. Your percent body fat is calculated based on equations. This technique provides body fat estimations similar to underwater weighing, though more data is needed on competitive athletes. The subject sits in an enclosed capsule (Bod Pod) while a computer measures the amount of air displaced. This is an expensive system, but is less inconvenient than underwater weighing. However, this technique may not be widely available.

Bioelectrical Impedance Analysis (BIA)

Use of bioelectrical impedance has markedly increased over the past ten years because it is relatively inexpensive, portable, and convenient. BIA is based on the conductive property of different tissues within the body. Because muscles contain a high percentage of water, they conduct current more quickly than fat stores. This machine passes a small and undetectable current through the body and analyzes the resistance to the flow of the current. The slower the signal, the more fat you have.

While BIA is relatively quick and simple, it may overestimate body fat in lean individuals, and results are affected by hydration levels. You should be well hydrated for the test but also not drink fluids four hours before the test to empty your bladder. It is best if you do not exercise within twelve hours of the test. Alcohol, diuretics, and caffeine should also be avoided prior to this measurement.

Many individuals are now purchasing a home scale (Tanita scale) that measures body fat with this technique. You should take the readings at the same time of day, be well hydrated, and have an empty bladder. Avoid early morning readings when you are most likely to be dehydrated.

Skinfold Calipers

The skinfold caliper method is the most widely used technique and the most inexpensive and convenient method for measuring body fat. A skilled technician uses calipers to indirectly measure the thickness of subcutaneous fat underneath the skin. Several standard skinfold sites have been identified on the body (abdomen, arm, thigh, hip area, and back of shoulder). They must be accurately marked, and the skinfold is then pinched and gently pulled away from the body. The sum of several skinfolds (anywhere from three to seven sites) is plugged into a formula.

This technique has several disadvantages. For one, it requires a skilled technician. This technique also assumes that subcutaneous fat is proportional to total body fat. Skinfold measurements may also underestimate body fat in lean athletes. It is also important that formulas appropriate for athletes and a specific sport are utilized when calculating body fat.

However, when kept in perspective, this technique can be reliable and accurate. When this technique is utilized, you can calculate not only the percent fat but also obtain a number that is the sum of all the skinfolds measured. This absolute number is not formula dependent and can be monitored over time. For example, a thirty-year-old male endurance athlete may have a three-site skinfold sum of 40 millimeters and estimated body fat of 12 percent. A follow-up measurement at several months may show an increase in body weight and a skinfold sum of 36 millimeters. These results would indicate a probable loss in body fat and increase in muscle mass. This trend can be monitored over a month or year's time, providing useful feedback regarding training and diet. Tape measure readings can also be combined with skinfold assessment. Measurements are taken at thigh, arm, and abdominal sites.

LOSING BODY FAT

Because your body composition is the result of genetics as well as training and diet, some athletes may fall naturally at an optimal body composition while others may struggle due to hereditary factors. Extreme efforts to maintain a set body composition may not be worth the energy, as intense weight loss approaches may compromise the quality of your diet and training. It is also important to keep a perspective on body fat. Aim for a healthy and appropriate range rather than a specific number. Body fat levels may also change over the course of a season depending on the phase of your training and the stage of your competitive career.

If you are considering improving your body fat composition, have it assessed by a skilled technician. An optimal goal weight can be determined, but it is important to be realistic regarding how much body fat you want to lose and how quickly you should reach your goal. This may require some professional advice and realism on your part.

First you should consider your genetics. Experts suggest that 25 to 40 percent of the fat our body stores is related to our genetics. If you have a history of struggling with weight loss and maintenance, or the same can be said of your family members, you should consider a moderate and gentle weight loss goal. Next look at your lifestyle. Food choices are heavily influenced by your schedule, commitments, environment, and stress levels. It is important for your weight loss goals to be reasonable, as you not only have to meet the energy demands of training but life and work as well.

Dieting Pitfalls

Dieting certainly presents several pitfalls for the endurance athlete. An athlete who is glycogen depleted, electrolyte depleted, low on protein, and dehydrated from dieting will not perform at her best, and likely will perform poorly. Rigid dieting and too much calorie restriction can deplete body fuel stores. Intense weight loss efforts can also result in hormonal imbalances, iron deficiency anemia, compromised bone health, and loss of muscular power. Severe dieting can also make you crabby and tired. Dieting just isn't fun.

Food is fuel for your hard-working body, and your body does not respond positively when fuel runs low. A low fuel gauge sends out a slew of appetite triggering brain chemicals that drive you to eat. What many dieters perceive as a lack of will power is really the body's drive for self-preservation. Restricting foods can lead to overeating and even binge-eating, thwarting weight loss efforts. Besides playing games with the body, dieting wreaks havoc with the mind. Restrictive eating can lead to feelings of deprivation and a preoccupation with food.

Besides triggering overeating, drastic calorie reduction can break down body protein stores for energy. This muscle loss not only hinders your strength and power, but also negatively impacts your metabolism. Muscle is what keeps your furnace burning. Your body also responds to calorie restriction by lowering its resting metabolic rate. Eating normally can restore your metabolism, though this may be difficult if you have a history of repeated dieting. Over time your body may become more efficient at utilizing calories and storing body fat.

Healthy Weight Loss Guidelines

Healthy weight loss starts with setting a realistic goal and avoiding quick, unbalanced, and extreme weight loss approaches. Try to accomplish a realistic weight loss in a reasonable amount of time and at an "off-season" time of year. Let's take a look at some sensible weight loss guidelines.

- **Set a realistic calorie deficit.** Women should not exceed a weight loss of one pound weekly, and men two pounds weekly, especially during heavy training periods. Losing one pound weekly requires a deficit of 500 calories daily. Greater weight loss requires even more restriction. Losing two pounds weekly requires a 1,000-calorie deficit, clearly calling for some intense calorie cutting and calorie burning efforts. Trimming no more than 200–300 calories daily may be the safest and most effective long-term weight loss approach. This mild reduction should have no metabolism lowering effects and will not precipitate feelings of hunger and deprivation.

- **Keep a food journal to assess your current eating habits.** Write down your food intake, times eaten, and portions for one week. Record your training times in conjunction with your food intake. You can also record your moods, thoughts, and feelings that correlate with your food intake to determine some of your eating triggers such as stress or fatigue. Assess your intake. Make sure that you are following the principles of post-exercise recovery nutrition. Monitor your hunger and fullness patterns. Do you often wait until you are ravenous before eating? Do you get overfull at meals? Do you eat for comfort or in reaction to stress fairly often? Do you have significant drops in your energy levels during the day? You may be surprised at how much you actually consume during the day. Writing your food intake down can also be very helpful in keeping you on track while you are trying to lose weight, as it makes you accountable and conscious of your food choices.

- **Have a strategy or plan for reducing your caloric intake.** There are a number of effective ways to reduce your caloric intake. It is important that you eat well post-exercise, and practice the recovery nutrition guidelines reviewed. If you eat out frequently you may be consuming too much hidden fat in your diet. Other techniques for reducing fat intake include choosing leaner meats, switching to low fat dairy products, minimizing added fats and those used in cooking, and decreasing the frequency of sweets. You can also cut back on high calorie fluids. Alcohol is an obvious choice, as are sodas and juices. Pay attention to portions when you eat out or grab items on the run. A bagel or muffin can easily provide more than 300 calories.

Recovering from an Injury

At some point in your athletic career it is possible that you may experience some type of injury from strain, abrasions, bruising, and fractures. Most likely the speed at which your injury heals is of major concern to you. While you may have a rehabilitation program mapped out, the nutritional guidelines that you should follow while injured may not be as clear.

Nutritional considerations can vary among specific situations and individuals. But often during rehabilitation there is a natural fear of putting on body fat. Injury often results in significant changes in energy expenditure, as a result of a decrease from your usual training volume and intensity. When you are accustomed to consuming a significant amount of food, it may be difficult to know how and when to cut back on your caloric intake to achieve the proper caloric balance.

Muscle mass may also decrease when you are injured, depending on the type of rehabilitation program prescribed. Depending on the type and extent of the injury, caloric expenditure may decrease by several thousand calories per week. An athlete who decreases his training volume by four hours a week could experience a weekly one-pound weight gain if he kept up with his usual eating habits.

Regardless of the type of injury, it is important to eat nutritiously during this time. Injured athletes can keep a food record and determine their normal caloric intake. They then can trim anywhere from 200 to 500 calories or more daily to prevent weight gain. Often carbohydrate and protein amounts need to be decreased slightly to prevent a gain in body fat. Excess dietary fat that was easily burned off in training should also be shaved down. But avoid drastic dietary restrictions so that you don't miss out on needed nutrients. Often, some personalized guidance from a sports nutritionist can be helpful when you are injured.

If appropriate, a good resistance rehabilitation program provides a big calorie advantage. Building muscle takes work and energy, allowing you to consume more calories and somewhat offset the decreased caloric expenditure from training. If these weight training sessions are intense, consuming carbohydrates during training can facilitate recovery and muscle repair.

When you are injured, increasing your intake of certain nutrients and perhaps even supplementation may support the healing process. One of the principal functions of vitamin C is collagen synthesis. Collagen is required for the formation and maintenance of connective tissue such as cartilage, tendon, and bone. Vitamin C also plays a role in red blood cell synthesis. Load up on some good vitamin C sources as listed in Chapter 3. Fruits and vegetables are abundant in vitamin C and are also lower calorie foods. Increasing your intake of fruits and vegetables will also provide antioxidants and bioflavonoids that can protect your muscles against damage during exercise and support the healing process.

Food choices that can decrease inflammation may also be useful for related injuries. The guidelines outlined in Chapter 2 for increasing intake of alpha-linolenic acid and reducing intake of linoleic acid should be reviewed.

Zinc is also an important component of many enzymes involved in energy metabolism and is required for protein synthesis and wound healing. Good sources of zinc include lean red meat, turkey, milk, yogurt, and seafood—especially oysters. Zinc from animal protein is best absorbed. ■

- **Plan ahead.** Preparing meals ahead of time can help you avoid fatty restaurant foods. You can also pack healthy snacks such as fresh fruits and vegetables. Programming your food environment for success will go a long way to supporting your weight loss goals.

- **Eat balanced meals at the right times.** Having real meals will leave you feeling satisfied. Make sure that you consume meals throughout the day so you don't set yourself up for periods of intense hunger. Make sure that you have a full breakfast and lunch, and don't consume all your calories in the evening. Your body works best on a steady supply of fuel throughout the day.

- **Have some protein and fat with your meals and snacks.** These foods will keep you feeling full longer and help prevent hunger that can lead to an unplanned trip to the vending machine. Of course, choose lean proteins and small amounts of healthy fats. Look at your food journal to determine what times of day you get too hungry. Add a bit more protein or fat to the preceding meal or snack if hunger sets in quickly at specific times.

GAINING MUSCLE MASS

In contrast to athletes attempting to lose weight, others are focused on increasing muscle mass. Just as some individuals struggle to reach body fat goals, those with slender frames may struggle to achieve the ideal muscle-bound body. To achieve an increase in muscle mass, athletes often make resistance training part of their exercise program during their off-season. Muscle building can increase your strength-to-weight ratio and ultimately strength and power.

The most important nutrition guideline for building muscle is to consume enough calories. It takes energy to build body tissue, and inadequate amounts will impair your rate of muscle building. Often the perception is that these extra calories should come from protein. Although protein is required to build muscle tissue, this is only a small portion of the tissue building process. In fact, the amounts of protein that you require as an endurance athlete are more than adequate to cover your needs for muscle building.

Besides providing your body with enough energy to build tissue, you also need to provide your body with enough energy to perform resistance exercise. Inadequate carbohydrates required to fuel training will impair how quickly you build lean body mass. An additional 350–400 calories daily are needed to gain one pound of muscle mass per week. Because muscle glycogen is a significant fuel source during training, it would make sense that some of these additional calories come from carbohydrates.

Research has demonstrated that a hard weight training session depletes about 30 percent of your muscle glycogen stores and 30 percent of your muscle triglyceride stores, and also has a high reliance on the creatine phosphate energy system for fuel. While this may not sound significant, glycogen depletion is specific to muscles that you exercise and stress. The muscles you are specifically trying to develop may be completely depleted. If you wish to continue your aerobic training and resistance training again later in the week, your muscle glycogen stores need to be replenished with an adequate intake of carbohydrates.

Food sources should also provide plenty of protein, and you should not require any special supplements for muscle building. However, you should also consider practicing recovery nutrition after a strenuous resistance training sessions, just as you would after endurance exercise. Carbohydrates and a small amount of protein consumed after resistance training should work to stimulate muscle glycogen synthesis. This form of supplementation increases blood levels of insulin and growth hormone, both of which are tissue building agents. High glycemic carbohydrates can be emphasized after resistance training, just as they can after endurance exercise. Fluids should also be replaced, though dehydration may not be as marked as during endurance exercise.

In addition to taking carbohydrates after training, consuming carbohydrates during resistance exercise may also be beneficial. These training sessions can dip into muscle glycogen stores and utilize blood glucose for fuel. Sports drinks will also provide hydration and maintain blood glucose levels during these sessions. This nutrition strategy may be especially helpful if you have not eaten for several hours before the next filling meal. You can alternate consumption of these drinks with consumption of plenty of water. Eating some carbohydrates and small amounts of protein before exercise may also be beneficial. This pre-exercise meal provides the body with the fuel required for training and contributes to the overall nutrition goal of increasing protein synthesis and decreasing protein breakdown.

To gain muscle mass while following a strength training program requires an additional 350–400 calories daily, mainly from carbohydrates and some protein. Some strategies for obtaining additional calories include:

- Adding a bit more protein to sandwiches and dinners.
- Topping carbohydrate foods such as bagels with jams and honeys.
- Adding another snack to your meal plan.
- Adding a fruited yogurt, fruit smoothie, low fat shake, or instant breakfast drink to your meal plan.
- Adding a pasta or rice salad to your lunch.
- Considering a high calorie shake or meal replacement.
- Making oatmeal and soups with milk.
- Adding wheat germ, sunflower seeds, and dried fruit to cereals.
- Choosing higher calorie juices such as apple, cranberry, nectars, and blends.
- Choosing calorie dense cereals like muesli, granola, and Grape-Nuts.
- Having starchy vegetables like peas, corn, and winter squash.

THE SPECTRUM OF DISORDERED EATING

Endurance training and competition involves moving your body over a given distance for a set amount of time as quickly as possible. So having a lower level of body fat is considered to be a mechanical advantage. However, many athletes do become overly focused on their weight and body fat levels. Because athletes may be obsessive by nature, as well as perfectionistic and very competitive, some of these qualities may manifest in unrealistic weight and body fat goals, placing a high degree of importance on losing a few pounds. Pressure to lose this weight may come from a number of outside sources including trainers, coaches, and athletic peers. Being female also places an athlete at risk of being dissatisfied with body image.

Often, behavior that begins as an attempt to lose weight takes on a life of its own and develops into unhealthy groups of behaviors known as disordered eating. Disordered eating represents a full spectrum of eating behaviors with poor eating habits at one end and full-blown anorexia nervosa and bulimia nervosa at the other end. While full-blown eating disorders are not exceptionally high in most sports, studies indicate a high prevalence of disordered eating behavior and distorted concerns regarding body weight, body fat, and body shape among athletes. Some common disordered eating behaviors may include skipping meals, constant weighing, eating very little fat, and a fear that specific foods may promote unwanted weight gain. Binge eating, as characterized by consuming large amounts of food while feeling out of control, can be part of disordered eating.

Another term, anorexia athletica, describes a syndrome characterized by disordered eating and compulsive exercising. It is associated with an intense fear of gaining weight, despite being at normal or below normal weight, and is characterized by food restriction and excessive exercise. Binging, self-induced vomiting, and use of laxative and diuretics may also occur. Some athletes are able to stop these behaviors when participation in a sport stops. But for other athletes, this behavior develops into a full clinical eating disorder. Because of the various methodologies utilized, the prevalence of eating disorders measured among athletes has ranged from 1 percent to as high as 39 percent.

Eating disorders are complicated and multifactorial. Psychological and emotional issues such as anxiety and depression, an inability to cope with family and personal problems, life stresses, biochemical imbalances, and the pressure to be thin from both sport and society may be involved. Some triggers associated with

Nutrition for Pregnancy and Exercise

Many pregnant female athletes desire to maintain a high degree of fitness during pregnancy and often return to training and competition as quickly as possible. While you may be most concerned about consuming an adequate number of calories and appropriate weight gain, what you consume while planning a pregnancy is also very important.

Often women plan to see their physician before trying to conceive and take a prenatal multivitamin mineral supplement in order to obtain folic acid and other important nutrients. Folate (found from food sources) and folic acid (from supplement sources) deserve serious attention from women even contemplating pregnancy. An adequate intake of folate, both prior to conception and during the first several weeks of pregnancy, can help prevent birth defects such as spina bifida. Folate is used for the synthesis of DNA, the building block of all cells. During the first twenty-eight days of pregnancy, cells divide rapidly and form the neural tubes that become the baby's brain and spine. Many Americans fall short of the recommended 400 micrograms of folate. Good food sources include asparagus, lentils, spinach and other leafy green vegetables, dried beans such as kidney beans, and orange juice. Grain products such as bread, pasta, rice, and enriched flour are now being fortified with folic acid. Many health experts also recommend that any woman who may become pregnant take a multivitamin providing 400 micrograms of folate.

During the first three months of pregnancy, it is normal to have 0–5 pounds weight gain. After the first trimester, a weight gain of up to one pound weekly is normal. Generally a total weight gain of 25–35 pounds is recommended. Underweight or lean women may be advised to gain more, or about 28–40 pounds. Adequate weight gain comes down to finding the right balance of calories to build your own tissue during pregnancy, to support the growth of the baby, and to meet your energy needs from exercise in order to prevent having a low birth weight baby or a premature delivery. Starting in the second trimester, pregnancy requires only an additional 300 calories daily above your usual energy needs and another 10–12 grams of protein. These additional nutrient amounts are easily met with an increased food intake, with one example being 8 ounces of milk and a small turkey sandwich.

The expectant mother's weight gain comes from growth in her own body tissues, the baby's body weight, and tissues that support the baby's growth. It includes an increased blood volume, body fluid, breast tissue, and weight gain from the placenta, umbilical cord, and amniotic fluid. Your body stores fat in anticipation of lactation, which requires at least an additional 500 calories daily above your normal non-pregnancy requirements. Your physician will not only monitor your total weight gain, but also the pattern of your weight gain to make sure that it is appropriate.

Fluid requirements also increase when you are pregnant, and it is critical to maintain proper hydration when you train. Your basic fluid requirements are about 2.5–3 quarts daily, plus what you sweat during exercise. It is essential that you begin exercise well hydrated. Overheating could have serious negative effects on the unborn baby. Consume plenty of fluids several hours before exercise and drink at least 4–8 ounces of fluid every 15–20 minutes. You may also want to focus on consuming carbohydrates several

(continued on page 162)

(continued from page 161)

hours before exercise to prevent hypoglycemia. You can continue to ingest sports drinks, carbohydrate gels, and energy bars during exercise to maintain blood glucose levels, but avoid products that contain additional vitamins and minerals and any herbal ingredients. Your food choices and prenatal vitamin and mineral supplement should be more than adequate to meet your requirements. Herbal products have not been tested in pregnancy and should be avoided.

Other important nutrients to include in your diet during pregnancy are iron and calcium. Your iron requirements double due to your expanded blood volume. Most pregnant women receive adequate iron in their prenatal vitamin and mineral supplement, but some require an additional iron supplement in order to prevent anemia. Anemia can result in fatigue, shortness of breath, and increased delivery risks. The baby also runs the risk of developing anemia if your iron stores run too low. As an endurance athlete you may already have low iron stores. Your physician should check your iron levels early in pregnancy and at regular intervals afterward. Concentrate on including plenty of high iron foods in your diet, as listed in Chapter 3.

Calcium plays an important role in every woman's health and deserves extra attention during pregnancy. Your calcium requirements increase to 1,200 milligrams daily. As your baby builds bone, your bones serve as a calcium source. If your diet is inadequate to replenish this calcium reservoir, you run the risk of developing osteoporosis later in life. High calcium food sources are reviewed in Chapter 3. You may also want to consider taking a separate calcium supplement during pregnancy to meet your elevated requirements.

There are also certain nutrients and foods you should limit during pregnancy. Excess vitamin A intake from supplementation can increase risk of birth defects. Make sure you do not take a supplement that exceeds 5,000 IU of vitamin A daily. There is also no room for alcohol in your diet, as it can produce severe negative effects on the baby such as fetal alcohol syndrome. Caffeine should be restricted to no more than 300 milligrams daily or avoided altogether. Avoid saccharin and limit other artificial sweeteners as much as possible. Limit soft cheese such as Brie, Camembert, blue cheese, and feta cheese as they can increase your risk of bacterial contamination. In general, be careful with food safety. Never eat raw fish, and make sure that all meats are well cooked. Avoid any unpasteurized milk products and raw eggs. Fish can also be contaminated with polychlorinated biphenyls (PCBs) and mercury. Avoid fatty fish such as swordfish, mackerel, shark, bluefish, and striped bass. Limit canned tuna to less than 4 ounces weekly, and keep your total fish intake to 9–12 ounces weekly. Eat low fat fish and trim excess fat as much as possible. Avoid all herbal supplements and herbal products such as teas, as they have not been tested in pregnancy.

Lactation or breast-feeding increases your daily energy needs (from non-pregnancy requirements) to about 500 calories daily. Fat stores accumulated during pregnancy also serve as an important energy source for lactation. Your fluid needs are also high during this time. Weight loss can occur gradually with lactation, but it is best to try not to lose more than one pound weekly, as an overly restrictive diet will decrease the quantity of milk that you produce. Maintain your high calcium and iron intakes from pregnancy, and you can consider continuing to take your prenatal multivitamin mineral supplement. Continue to limit alcohol and caffeine as they can enter breast milk. It may be best to nurse before exercise due to transient changes that occur in breast milk with exercise. ■

eating disorders in athletes include traumatic life events such as relationship problems, recommendations to lose weight, prolonged periods of dieting, and a large discrepancy between actual weight and a self-defined ideal weight. It is possible that individuals at high risk for eating disorders may gravitate toward certain sports, but being involved in a sport may also trigger the eating disorder in a susceptible athlete. Table 7.1 describes some of the signs and symptoms of anorexia nervosa and bulimia nervosa.

There are several common warning signs that may signal the start of an eating disorder. They include repeatedly expressing concerns about body weight, refusal to

---

EATING DISORDERS

ANOREXIA NERVOSA

- Resistance to maintaining body weight at or above a minimally normal weight
- Intense fear of gaining weight or becoming fat even though underweight
- Distortion in the way in which one's body weight or shape is experienced; denial of the seriousness of current low body weight
- Infrequent or absent menstrual periods in females who have reached puberty

Physical Characteristics of Anorexia Nervosa

- Hair loss and growth of fine body hair
- Low pulse rate
- Sensitivity to cold
- Stress fractures, osteopenia, or osteoporosis
- Overuse injuries
- Abnormal fatigue
- Gastrointestinal problems

BULIMIA NERVOSA

- Recurrent episodes of binge eating, characterized by a sense of lack of control and by an excessive amount of food within a short period of time
- Purging behavior such as self-induced vomiting, misuse of laxatives, diuretics, enemas, or other medications
- Binge eating and purging behavior occur on average at least twice weekly for three months
- Self-esteem is inappropriately influenced by body shape and weight

Physical Characteristics of Bulimia Nervosa

- Frequent weight fluctuations
- Difficulty swallowing and throat damage
- Swollen glands
- Damaged tooth enamel from gastric acid
- Electrolyte imbalances and dehydration
- Menstrual irregularities
- Diarrhea or constipation

maintain even a minimal weight, periods of severe calorie restriction, and excessive physical activity that is not part of a balanced training program. Other warning signs may include food rituals, self-induced vomiting, and abuse of laxatives and diet pills. Many of these behaviors by themselves do not prove the presence of an eating disorder, but they justify further attention to the possible presence of a problem.

An athlete with an eating disorder requires the help of a team of skilled professionals trained in treating this condition. This should include a team of a physician, dietitian, and psychologist or therapist.

7.1

EATING DISORDERS

EATING DISORDER NOT OTHERWISE SPECIFIED

This category includes disorders of eating that do not meet the criteria for a specific eating disorder.

- Binge-eating disorder and episodes of binge eating without the use of compensatory behavior as seen in bulimia nervosa.
- Repeatedly chewing and spitting out, but not swallowing large amounts of food.
- The criteria for anorexia nervosa are met except that the frequency of binge eating and purging behavior occur less than twice weekly and for less than three months.
- All of the criteria for bulimia nervosa are met except that the individual has regular menstrual periods.
- Regular purging behaviors occur after consuming small amounts of food.

ANOREXIA ATHLETICA

This term has been used to describe a condition that is not a full-blown eating disorder.

- Characterized by disordered eating and compulsive exercising.
- Intense fear of weight gain despite weighing below the expected weight for age and height.
- Weight loss is achieved by food restrictions and extensive compulsive exercise.
- May involve self-induced vomiting, and abuse of laxatives and diuretics.

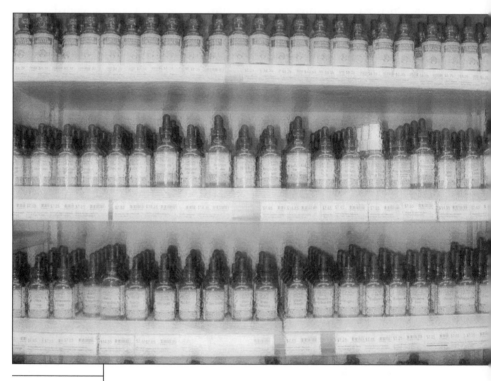

DON KARLE PHOTO

chapter **8**

NUTRITIONAL ERGOGENIC AIDS

Separating Fact from Fiction

"Gain 30 pounds of solid muscle in just 12 weeks. Too good to be true? Think again."

"How about an exclusive natural product for increasing endurance and fat loss without dangerous side effects? It has been clinically shown to increase metabolism and fat loss up to 48 percent without exercise."

SALES AND MARKETING OF ERGOGENIC AIDS

With sales estimated at $5.3 billion in 1999 and expected to increase to $7.2 billion in 2004, athletes have clearly embraced sports nutrition products as an important component of their training programs. Previous chapters have outlined practical uses for products such as sports drinks, gels, and bars, and high carbohydrate and meal replacement supplements that are backed by both research and the practical experience of elite athletes. Using these products knowledgeably and appropriately carries minimal risk (perhaps a bit of GI intolerance for some) and clear performance benefits (see Table 5.5).

However, there is another group of nutritional supplements that is aggressively marketed to athletes. Referred to as nutritional ergogenic aids, these products promise an extra performance edge. Nutritional ergogenic aid sales are a serious and lucrative business. Sales from one such product, creatine, skyrocketed from

$30 million in 1995 to $400 million in 2001. Dietary supplement sales for 2001 were $17.74 billion, including vitamins, herbs, minerals, sports nutrition products, and meal replacement products. Sales are estimated to exceed $20 billion by 2004.

Ergogenic aid sales are also a serious business for athletes. It is important that when you ingest a product in the quest for top performance you have verified that it is legal, effective, and safe. Unfortunately, many of these products are backed solely by strong and enticing claims, anecdotal hearsay, high-profile athlete and coach testimonials, and referenced "research" that has not been published in full in a reputable scientific journal. In reality, the majority of these supplements have not been thoroughly and appropriately tested. And many supplements that are tested independently of the manufacturers who supply them don't live up to their performance claims. But despite this lack of plausibility, it can be tempting to top off all your hard work with an easily ingested supplement that promises a quick and effective performance boost.

The term ergogenic means "to produce work." Nutritional ergogenic aids can increase physical power or energy production, enhance mental strength, or provide a mechanical edge. For example, it is claimed that several ergogenic aids enhance fat burning and provide fuel during exercise, caffeine may provide central nervous stimulation at the end of a race, and losing body fat provides a mechanical edge as it makes hill running or climbing during cycling easier.

With new products coming out monthly, athletes need to be discerning when evaluating nutritional ergogenic aids or performance enhancers. It is important to make knowledgeable choices about these products. This includes:

- Understanding how the ergogenic aid purportedly functions.
- Knowing the summary of the current research support on the supplement.
- Being aware of any safety concerns surrounding the product.
- Knowing if the product is a legal supplement for athletes.

Chances are you may try a supplement because it is widely talked about in your training group or surrounded by enticing marketing claims. It may also seem that with all the hard work, time, and money that you invest in your training, it is only logical that you give yourself every little legal performance edge possible. After all, you don't get up to train at 6:00 a.m. because you feel like goofing around. But taking supplements that you don't really need could be a waste of your time and especially your money. It is also important that the product (however effective) not endanger your health in any way. Finally, you do not want to inadvertently take a product that is illegal and be banned from competition due to a positive drug test.

Regulation of Dietary Supplement and Nutritional Ergogenic Aids

Athletes are bombarded with claims of the magical effects of nutritional ergogenic aids on performance. Advertising and claims surrounding these products have increased exponentially since the Dietary Supplement Health and Education Act (DSHEA) was passed in 1994. DSHEA significantly changed how all dietary supplements such as vitamins, minerals, herbs, amino acids, metabolites, and even hormones were tested, marketed, labeled, and manufactured.

From its inception, DSHEA generated much controversy as to whom it has really benefited, the consumer or the supplement industry. But one thing is clear, even as interpretation of the DSHEA regulations continue to evolve and are tested by various manufacturers, consumers need to be informed regarding dietary supplements, and athletes need to be informed regarding ergogenic aids.

Unlike regulation of a drug or food additive, supplement manufacturers are not required to prove that a dietary supplement works. Under DSHEA, manufacturers are responsible for making sure that products are safe. The government does not review these products before they are put on the market, but the Food and Drug Administration (FDA) can take action against any unsafe dietary supplement products. However, the FDA cannot evaluate the thousands of products on the market, and makes selective use of time and resources. It is more likely that they will respond only to products that have resulted in significant adverse health effects that occur on a large scale.

You may also notice on the label a somewhat loosely defined "nutrition support claim." These claims may relate to the "structure and function" of the body and "general well being." While a certain set of conditions must be met to make these claims, they do not require prior FDA approval. Manufacturers must be able to substantiate that the claim is "truthful and not misleading," but cannot promise to prevent or cure a disease. Some nutrition support claims may include "maintains a healthy circulatory system," or "helps maintain a healthy intestinal flora." Note that supplements providing these types of claims must also state: "This product is not intended to diagnose, treat, cure, or prevent any disease."

The FDA also recommends that the discerning consumer realizes that it is up to each company to decide how their manufacturing practices will prepare and package supplements, thereby affecting their purity, safety, potency, and overall quality. According to the FDA, a consumer can contact the manufacturer and request product safety information and research support, preferably not in-house published data. They can also question if the firm has a quality control system in place and if any adverse event reports have resulted from use of their product.

You should also review the "Supplement Facts" label on the package of dietary supplements. Unlike conventional foods, the dosage on labels is not standardized. So remember that higher amounts than needed or are safe may be recommended. The label will provide the following:

- Statement of identity—Ginseng
- Net quantity of ingredients—60 capsules
- A structure-function claim statement—Increases energy
- Directions for use—Take one capsule daily
- Supplement Facts Label—Serving size, amount, active ingredient

- Other ingredients listed in descending order of predominance by common name or proprietary blend
- Name and address of packer, manufacturer, or distributor

Unfortunately, even if companies are accused and fined regarding false claims on dietary supplements, they may not de deterred from promoting new products. Often fines may be rendered insignificant by a large volume of sales generated while claims are investigated.

Evaluating Ergogenic Aids

Is It Effective?

Valid scientific testing of a nutritional ergogenic aid costs time, money, and resources. Tests of a supplement's effect upon performance should be conducted with elite or well-trained athletes. For these and other reasons, much of the supplement industry forgoes testing and relies heavily on testimonials, anecdotes, and untested scientific theories rather than research studies to promote their products. But a theory is not proof. A theory is a hypothesis or intriguing idea that requires testing. "Scientific breakthroughs" may be new and interesting ideas with little or no basis in fact.

A scientific trial remains the best way in which to examine the effectiveness of ergogenic aids on performance. Here, athletes' experiences can be helpful to researchers, who desire to focus on potentially effective substances. Scientists can use them to determine what products are worth testing and what dosages are appropriate for test protocols. Testing should closely mimic real athletic performance conditions. Researchers should control for age, level of training, and nutritional status. Various dosages, supplementation periods, types of exercise, and performance testing may need to be incorporated.

Studies should control for the placebo effect as much as possible by incorporating a double-blind design. Subjects receive both the substance being tested and a placebo. To minimize bias, subjects and researchers don't know which product is being administered when. In addition to a placebo trial, there may be a control (no treatment) group. These are only some of the needed features of well-designed testing that satisfy the scientist, but not always the athlete. A large change in performance is required for outcomes to be considered statistically significant. In many cases, however, changes produced by nutritional supplementation are likely to be smaller. While a 1- to 3-percent change may not be statistically adequate, it could be useful in elite competitions where outcomes can come down to fractions of seconds. Researchers also report the overall performance effect within a group. Positive results of individuals within a group may be diluted by the negative or neutral responses of other subjects. Not all subjects respond in the same way to a particular substance.

Unfortunately, even well-designed studies can be quoted out of context. Research findings are extrapolated to inappropriate conclusions. Companies often state that they are in the process of conducting research. Other times they say that research is "in-house" or has simply never been published in reputable peer-reviewed journals. And even well-designed preliminary studies require verification through additional sound research. Unfortunately, even studies published in reputable journals can provoke criticism when placed under close scrutiny. Additionally, patented nutritional ergogenic aids may also look impressive, yet patents are not granted based on the effectiveness of the product but rather on its distinguishable differences. Patents can be obtained with a theoretical model rather than objective double-blind research.

Is It Safe?

False claims aside, the next step in determining if you should use an ergogenic aid is evaluating safety concerns. As previously mentioned, supplement manufacturers are not required to prove a product's safety. Negative effects from products may be acute, mild, or temporary, but they can also be serious and chronic. Some dietary supplements may be toxic or decrease the absorption of other nutrients, especially in high doses where the "more is better" belief prevails. Ironically, independent testing has also found that many supplements do not contain the ingredients marked on the label. Often products are watered down or contain other unlisted ingredients that may be harmful or illegal.

Is It Legal?

As a competitive athlete, particularly if you may be drug-tested, you do not want to inadvertently take a dietary supplement that contains a banned substance. The past several years has seen a significant increase in the number of positive tests at the elite and professional level, claimed to be the result of a contaminated or misla-beled dietary supplement. All athletic governing bodies have some regulation regarding the use of ergogenic aids. Even if you avoid these banned products, such as Ma Huang or androstenodione, reading labels is not a 100-percent guarantee of avoiding banned products. Cross contamination can occur in the manufacturing process, and the purity of these supplements is often questioned.

Specific nutritional ergogenic aids can benefit athletes under certain conditions. However, the supplement industry is an extremely profitable business that relies on theories and testimonials to market products. Ergogenic aid theories may even be extrapolated from clinical research on disease states or nutrient deficiencies. To say that this product will then produce a performance improvement is not a scientific breakthrough, but a leap in logic. Even with proven ergogenic aids it is important to keep their role in perspective. While they may produce small performance improve-ments, ergogenic aids are no substitute for proper training, nutrition, and psycho-logical preparation.

POPULAR NUTRITIONAL ERGOGENIC AIDS

Research Support, Safety, and Practical Issues

This section will review several popular nutritional ergogenic aids for scientific valid-ity as determined by quality research. Any safety concerns and any practical issues regarding use of these supplements will also be reviewed in this section. Not surprisingly, many sports physiologists and sports nutritionists do not demonstrate overwhelming support for the majority of these supplements. They would rather that you train and eat properly! Ultimately, whether or not you take a supplement is your decision. But it should be an informed decision and a safe one. If you do choose to try a supplement with little scientific backing, do not exceed the dose and duration tested.

Energy Systems and Ergogenic Aids

The three energy or power systems were briefly reviewed in Chapter 4. They are the ATP creatine phosphate system; anaerobic glycolysis or lactic acid system; and the aerobic glycolytic and lipolytic systems. Many ergogenic aids are designed to enhance the power output of one of these systems. It is important that you appreciate what power systems are predominately utilized during your training and competition efforts. Perhaps you are taking a supplement designed to enhance a system that is not a significant part of your training program. Why take a supplement designed to enhance the creatine phosphagen system that supplies energy during short bursts of activity when your goal is steady state aerobic training? Some supplements do not affect an energy system, but may be thought of as performance enhancing as they can assist in fluid hyperhydration, such as in the case of glycerol, or are believed to enhance your immune system, like the amino acid glutamine.

Ergogenic Aids with Scientific Support

Bicarbonate

Sodium bicarbonate, commonly known as baking soda, is an alkaline salt thought to buffer the acid build-up in the muscle cells caused by training that stresses the anaerobic glycolysis or lactic acid energy system. During exercise that stresses the lactic acid system, acid accumulation inhibits muscle contraction and is associated with fatigue. The majority of both laboratory and field studies show that bicarbonate supplementation or "soda loading" improves performance in high intensity tasks, both continuous and intermittent, that last one to seven minutes. This effect appears to be moderate, specific to the athlete and the event, and basically should not be of great benefit to an endurance athlete.

Sodium bicarbonate appears to be safe when taken in the recommended dose of 140 milligrams per pound of body weight. For a 150-pound athlete this translates to a dose of 5 teaspoons of baking soda that provides 21,000 milligrams or 21 grams of bicarbonate. Safety, however, should not be confused with side effects. Baking soda should be consumed with plenty of water, about 1 quart, when taken one to two hours prior to exercise. This may or may not mitigate reported side effects in some individuals that include nausea, bloating, abdominal pain, and diarrhea. Only two studies have found that bicarbonate enhances endurance exercise lasting about one hour. Overall, this supplement is not likely to be of great benefit to the endurance athlete. Clearly, it must be determined in training if side effects may occur.

Caffeine

One of the oldest known drugs, caffeine belongs to a group of compounds known as methyl-xanthines. Caffeine is found naturally in coffee beans, tea leaves, cocoa beans, and cola nuts. Caffeine-containing foods are a natural part of many athletes' diets, including coffee, tea, chocolate and soft drinks. Many of these products provide 30–100 milligrams per serving, while some over-the-counter medications provide 100–200 milligrams per serving.

While it appears that caffeine does provide some muscle glycogen sparing effects, this appears to be limited to the first fifteen to twenty minutes of exercise. Researchers are not certain exactly how caffeine produces this effect. The classic theory is that caffeine elevates free fatty acids in the blood, which exercising muscles use for energy while conserving muscle glycogen. Caffeine may also impact the enzyme that breaks down glycogen. Besides sparing glycogen, caffeine also stimulates the central nervous system (increasing alertness), stimulates blood circulation and heart function and releases epinephrine, all of which could enhance a variety of performance-related functions. Caffeine also stimulates calcium release from the muscle, which stimulates muscular contraction.

Recent well-designed studies utilizing elite athletes have found that caffeine can effectively enhance performance when consumed in legal amounts. Doses as low as 1.5–2.0 milligrams per pound of weight are effective. The optimal dose appears to be 2.25–2.7 milligrams per pound. Consuming higher caffeine amounts can result in an athlete testing positive and provides no additional performance benefits. Currently, the International Olympic Committee regards a caffeine level of 12 micrograms per millimeter of urine as exceeding legal limits. While it is estimated that 800 milligrams of caffeine would be required to exceed legal limits, individuals may have "thresholds" that result in a positive test from lower levels. Most studies have had subjects ingest caffeine one hour prior to exercise.

It is important for you to appreciate that not all athletes react to caffeine in a similar manner. Some individuals may not have a performance response to caffeine, and some athletes experience negative side effects that include increased heart rate, muscle tremors, headaches, unsteadiness, nausea, and GI intolerance. Caffeine's diuretic effect has long been debated, but it appears that it is essentially insignificant. Studies indicate that caffeine does not increase urine output during exercise.

Athletes who wish to use caffeine as an ergogenic aid during competition should experiment during training. Many athletes choose to abstain from caffeine intake for several days before competition to enhance the effect of the pre-competition dose. Then appropriate doses of caffeine can be obtained from morning coffee or other caffeine-containing drinks. During ultraendurance exercise, many athletes also ingest cola drinks that contain caffeine. Practice this technique in training as well if you are considering this option during competition.

Creatine

With sales at $400 million in 2001, creatine is clearly a supplement that came out of the starting blocks and kicked into high gear. Fortunately, creatine is one of the best-researched ergogenic aids, making it possible for sports nutritionists to provide clear and confident recommendations regarding this sports nutrition supplement.

Creatine is often advertised as a steroid alternative, but it is really more comparable to glycogen loading. Just as carbohydrate ingestion maximizes glycogen content of the muscle, "creatine loading" can increase muscle creatine stores. Your normal intake of creatine is about 2 grams daily (perhaps less for vegetarians), and it is also synthesized in the liver and kidney. Creatine is an essential fuel of the ATP creatine phosphate system. Loading the muscle with creatine is designed to increase ATP resynthesis. This power system typically stores enough fuel to last six to ten seconds. Creatine can also buffer lactic acid and transport ATP to be utilized for muscle contraction.

Muscle biopsies have confirmed that rapid loading can be achieved with 25 grams of creatine daily divided into five to six doses. A more gentle loading protocol is 3 grams daily over twenty-eight days. Unlike carbohydrates, creatine appears to remain trapped in the muscle without supplementation for four to five weeks. About 30 percent of individuals who creatine load appear to be "non-responders." Ingesting about 75–100 grams of carbohydrates has been demonstrated to enhance creatine accumulation in the muscle. You should also be aware that a two- to five-pound weight gain is associated with creatine loading. Scientists believe this to be water gain, as urine output decreases during the loading phase. Though not documented in the scientific literature, anecdotal reports abound that creatine loading is associated with muscle cramping and GI upset.

We know that creatine ingestion can load the muscle, but how does it affect performance? Creatine loading appears to increase the rate of creatine resynthesis during recovery (twenty seconds to five minutes) from bouts of high intensity exercise (six to thirty seconds). Creatine loading delays fatigue during this type of activity, appears to benefit resistance training, and would be expected to support interval training. Improvements in performance during these types of training sessions may eventually improve your overall effectiveness as an endurance athlete, however, it does not appear to directly enhance endurance exercise. Research does not support that creatine would enhance an all-out sprint effort that could occur at the end of a race.

Endurance athletes should consider during which phase of their training program creatine loading would be most beneficial, perhaps during a heavy phase of resistance training. This may occur during the off-season for many endurance athletes. Creatine loading may also only be necessary once or twice yearly due to the cyclical nature of your training and to the muscle's ability to hold creatine for several weeks. Consume plenty of fluids if you creatine load and take it with carbohydrates to maximize muscle uptake. It is not recommended that you supplement for more than sixty days, and it should be at a low dose of 3 grams during this time period. Loading at 30 grams daily for five days, however, appears to be very effective. Creatine is currently legal. However, there have been some concerns of cross contamination of creatine products in recent years, as athletes ingesting this supplement have tested positive for banned prohormone products.

While creatine may have a place in the resistance training component of your program, this well-researched supplement may not have great significance for the endurance athlete. There is no substantial data to support that creatine loading offers any performance benefit during aerobic exercise.

Ergogenic Aids with Mixed Scientific Support

Branched Chain Amino Acids (BCAA)

Leucine, isoleucine, and valine are the three essential branched chain amino acids and can be obtained from a wide variety of foods. They are also located primarily in the muscle and can be used for energy during endurance exercise lasting longer than two hours when muscle carbohydrate stores run low. Proponents of BCAA supplementation maintain that they can prevent muscle breakdown during exercise, improve recovery after exercise when ingested post-exercise, and delay the mental fatigue or "brain drain" that can occur in the later stages of exercise when BCAA levels fall.

While the theory surrounding BCAAs is interesting, the research is far from con-clusive. Most well-controlled field studies and laboratory studies have reported no ergogenic effects with acute BCAA supplementation. One study that supplemented for fourteen days did find an improvement in a 40-kilometer time trial cycling per-formance. Subjects in one triathlon study did run faster, though it was not consid-ered statistically significant. Perhaps more research on ultraendurance exercise, dur-ing which BCAA would become a significant fuel source, is needed. But for now, consuming adequate carbohydrates and calories during exercise appears to be a good technique for preventing use of muscle mass as a fuel source during exercise. There is also no data to support that BCAA play a special role in muscle recovery after exercise. Rather, intake of mostly carbohydrates and lesser amounts of protein, as reviewed in Chapter 4, is very effective for post-exercise recovery.

The theory regarding prevention of mental fatigue with BCAA derives from the fact that as blood levels of BCAA fall during endurance exercise, levels of blood tryp-tophan increase, resulting in increased brain serotonin levels. Serotonin can pro-duce symptoms of sleepiness and fatigue. So in theory, BCAA supplementation could prevent serotonin levels in the brain from rising and prevent fatigue. It has been measured that you need to consume large amounts of BCAA to actually affect serotonin levels. Study doses ranged from 7 to 20 grams, though most packaged products come in smaller milligram units. Consuming these high doses is inconve-nient during exercise, and negative side effects include a bad taste in the mouth, ammonia build-up in the blood and muscle, and GI problems. Also, consuming adequate carbohydrates during exercise, a much more convenient strategy, is what is really needed to prevent your muscles from using BCAA for energy. Presently, the research does not substantiate this theory or BCAA supplementation.

Glutamine

Glutamine is an amino acid synthesized in the muscle tissue. It is the most abun-dant amino acid in the body and used as a fuel source by the cells of the immune system. Impaired glutamine status has been associated with the overtrained state in athletes. Overtrained athletes are thought to be more susceptible to upper respiratory tract infections and other infections.

Blood glutamine levels fall during endurance exercise and remain lowered during the recovery phase several hours after exercise. Glutamine depletion is thought to become cumulative if recovery between sessions is inadequate, as overtrained athletes have lower blood glutamine levels. However, adequate daily carbohydrate consumption is thought to possibly be the most effective means for preventing glutamine depletion.

The theory maintains that glutamine supplementation could help prevent the immune problems suffered by overtrained athletes. Research data, however, are not consistent in proving this true. Only one study has reported that supplementation reduced the incidence of infection the week following a heavy exercise session. What is likely is that glutamine supplementation benefits those athletes with a true deficiency and that it is not a general cure for immune system problems.

Glycerol

Glycerol is a colorless, liquid alcohol found naturally in fats and is produced from the breakdown of fat. Glycerol is available as a glycerine solution or as part of hyperhydration supplements for athletes. Use of glycerol is thought to be an effective means for hyperhydration before training and competition because it holds and attracts water like a sponge. If taken properly and with the correct amount of fluid, glycerol can hold about 36 ounces of fluid in the body. It may be useful for offsetting exercise in environments where sweat loss is so great that it cannot be fully replaced.

Study results are still mixed on glycerol hyperhydration. Several studies support that hyperhydration derived from glycerol ingestion can maintain lower heart rate and body core temperature during exercise in the heat. In turn, other studies found that glycerol hyperhydration exerted no beneficial physiological effect during endurance exercise.

When diluted and mixed property, glycerol appears relatively safe to use. Dosages used in research have been about 0.45 grams per pound of body weight, with each gram of solution diluted with three-fourths of an ounce of water. Glycerol solutions should be consumed one to two-and-a-half hours before exercise. You should be very careful if you want to experiment with glycerol. Some physiologists recommend that it be used under medical supervision only. Athletes who have experimented with glycerol have reported headaches, bloating, nausea, vomiting, and dizziness. Pregnant women or individuals with high blood pressure, diabetes, or kidney disease should not use glycerol due to potential negative side effects.

Glycerol hyperhydration supplements have been targeted toward endurance athletes. It may be appropriate for situations in which dehydration and excessive heat conditions are likely to occur. It may also be useful for rehydration in situations where quick recovery from fluid losses is required. Don't exceed the recommended amounts of glycerol, and experiment first with this product in training. Most glycerol-fluid mixtures should be taken ninety minutes to three hours before endurance competition. However, you still need to consume adequate amounts of fluid while competing when you take this supplement.

Ergogenic Aids Lacking Scientific Support

Arginine, Lysine, Ornithine

The amino acids arginine, lysine, and ornithine are often sold individually or in combination as "legal anabolic compounds" and "recovery agents." Claims surrounding these products include promoting release of growth hormone and a subsequent increase in lean body mass and decrease in body fat. These claims surfaced after two studies found that infusing these amino acids directly into the bloodstream stimulated the release of human growth hormone, which is involved in building muscle tissue.

However the effects of oral supplementation on human growth hormone are very questionable. Several well-controlled studies have verified that oral supplementation is not comparable to intravenous infusion. Other studies utilizing oral supplementation have been criticized for their design. One study that provided a large oral dose of arginine and ornithine found a slight increase in growth hormone release. However, this was most likely stimulated by the resistance training rather than the amino acid intake. High oral dosages of these amino acids are also associated with gastrointestinal problems.

Arginine, lysine, and ornithine are available individually or in mixtures in powder or tablet form. Dosages used in several research studies were 2 to 3 grams, and 6 grams may cause gastrointestinal distress. High doses of amino acids may also inhibit absorption of other amino acids. Doses used in several studies are also easily obtained by consuming high protein foods. Use of these supplements is unlikely to be beneficial.

Carnitine

Often promoted as a "metabolic fat-burner," carnitine is a non-essential nutrient formed in the liver from two amino acids. Your skeletal muscles contain at least 90 percent of the carnitine in your body. Carnitine is of interest to endurance athletes because it carries fat into the cells to be burned for energy during exercise. If carnitine supplementation did increase fat burning and decrease your body's reliance on glycogen and blood glucose, it could enhance performance.

Carnitine is unlikely to be an effective ergogenic aid, as carnitine supplementation does not appear to increase muscle carnitine levels (as measured by muscle biopsies). Glycogen sparing with carnitine supplementation was also not found in these studies. Only one study found a slight increase in muscle carnitine content after supplementation with 2 grams daily. Other studies found no improvements in exercise performance with carnitine supplementation. Two studies that did find a positive performance effect have been criticized for their methodology and design.

Carnitine supplementation appears to be safe if you consume the L-carnitine form of the nutrient only. DL-carnitine can be toxic, as it depletes L-carnitine and may lead to a deficiency. You can consume 2–4 grams daily for up to one month; 1- to 2-gram doses have been taken for six months.

Chromium

Chromium is a trace mineral often marketed as a legal alternative to anabolic steroids and human growth hormone. Scientists have long known that chromium enhances the effects of the hormone insulin, which regulates glucose metabolism. Adults with impaired glucose regulation have been measured to have positive responses with chromium supplementation. Insulin also promotes the uptake of amino acids into muscle cells and regulates protein metabolism. This protein building function has linked chromium to an increase in muscle mass.

Proponents of chromium supplementation for athletes maintain that many are chromium deficient and a supplement would improve protein building. Other proponents believe that high chromium doses could stimulate greater-than-normal muscle building. It has not been firmly established that athletes are chromium deficient. However, the North American diet is high in refined grains which may trigger a higher release of insulin and require more chromium in the diet than is normally consumed.

Studies on chromium supplementation have produced mixed, but mostly negative, results. The more recent and better designed studies monitored and controlled for exercise training and carefully measured body composition. These studies found no significant gains in muscle mass with chromium supplementation. Earlier studies that showed some positive results were not as carefully controlled. Higher doses of chromium in several studies have also not shown significant gains in muscle mass.

With high sales of chromium picolinate and large doses recommended by manufacturers, safety concerns have been raised. There is not much long-term data on chromium doses beyond 200 micrograms. Because chromium is a mineral, concern has been raised about large, chronic doses. Minerals often compete with one another for absorption, and one study did find that iron status was compromised with chromium supplementation.

Clearly, adequate chromium intake is important. Especially good sources are whole grain breads and cereals, mushrooms, asparagus, apples, raisins, cocoa, peanuts, peanut butter, and prunes. Various sports nutrition supplements such as recovery drinks and bars are often supplemented with chromium, and many regular multivitamin-mineral supplements also contain this mineral. Try not to exceed 200 micrograms daily from supplemental sources. Most diets do not exceed 50 micrograms of chromium daily.

Overall, chromium's ability to build muscle mass in athletes appears highly doubtful. Supplementation in safe doses is only appropriate to correct a deficiency and compensate for an inadequate diet.

Ginseng

Ginseng is a popular substance that has been used for thousands of years in Chinese medicine. Ginseng extracts contain several chemicals, the most important being glycosides or ginsenosides. There are various plant species and forms of ginseng.

Ginseng is considered to be an adaptogen, a term used to describe a substance that aids the body's response to stress and increases energy levels. This includes physical stress such as intense exercise. Numerous theories regarding how ginseng exerts this effect have been proposed, though the actual underlying mechanism has not been determined.

Many of the heavily marketed claims surrounding ginseng were on studies conducted in the 1960s and 1970s. Few of these studies were well-controlled, and most had many research design flaws. Seven more recent, well-controlled studies reported no significant effects on performance measures. Overall, the effects of ginseng have not been thoroughly researched.

Ginseng appears to be relatively safe when taken in doses recommended by the manufacturer. However, excessive use may result in high blood pressure, nervousness, and sleeplessness in some individuals. Ginseng is legal. Be wary of gingseng-containing products that may contain other substances such as ephedrine, which is banned.

Ginseng content in commercial products is also likely to be highly variable, and some preparations have been found not to contain detectable levels of ginsenosides.

Beta-Hydroxy-Beta-Methylbutarate (HMB)

HMB is primarily marketed to strength and power athletes and is one of the fastest-selling supplements on the market. Endurance athletes who weight train and want to facilitate muscle recovery may be interested in this supplement.

HMB is not actually a nutrient but is produced in small amounts when the amino acid leucine is metabolized. You produce only about 0.2–0.4 grams of HMB daily. HMB was first developed by scientists and then patented by the company that produces HMB and that has sponsored much of the research.

Much of the initial HMB research was done on animals, but there is also human data. Some of these studies have been published in full, and others currently only in abstract form. While some data has found greater increases in muscle mass and less markers of muscle damage, these studies did not always control for diet, which can have a significant impact upon muscle gain in conjunction with weight training. One well-controlled study found no ergogenic benefit from HMB supplementation.

Further published data on this supplement is needed. Currently HMB is legal. A daily dose of 3 grams also appears to be safe when taken for an eight-week period.

Medium Chain Triglycerides (MCTs)

MCTs have been available for clinical use for several years but have only recently been promoted to athletes. Because of their smaller size (compared to long-chain triglycerides), MCTs empty from the stomach more quickly and are more easily absorbed. In fact, they are absorbed as quickly as glucose and transported to the liver where they are metabolized. Their ergogenic benefit would result in providing quick fuel during exercise and sparing muscle glycogen during extended training.

Of the several studies conducted with MCT oil, one found a performance improvement, while the others did not. One study did determine that the amount of MCT oil that can be tolerated within the gastrointestinal tract might be limited. GI symptoms ranging from mild to severe can result. Consuming carbohydrates prior to exercise (as has been recommended in this book) could also negate the effects of MCT supplementation. Overall, this supplement is not recommended for endurance athletes.

Pyruvate

Pyruvate is commonly sold as DHAP, which is a combination of dihydroxyacetone and pyruvate. This supplement is promoted to improve endurance exercise, promote fat loss, and increase muscle mass.

Studies that have tested pyruvate on endurance performance need to be put in perspective. These studies used a small number of untrained subjects exercising at moderate intensity and may not have much relevance to endurance athletes. In addition, several of the study protocols utilized 25 grams of pyruvate combined with 75 grams of dihydroxyacetone. Many commercial preparations contain much smaller doses. However, these studies did measure an increase in endurance with the supplement.

Pyruvate does not appear to have much validity as a fat burner either. One often quoted study restricted participants to a 1,000 calorie daily diet and no activity. It would be impractical to apply this data to an endurance athlete.

Ribose

Ribose is hyped as a supplement that can improve muscle recovery, boost energy, enhance endurance, support cardiovascular fitness, and rebuild ATP. It is a sugar formed from the conversion of glucose, is considered the starting substance for ATP production, and is part of the metabolic pathway that results in ATP resynthesis.

However, published research on the effect of ribose in athletic performance is relatively limited. Ribose did benefit one group of men who suffered from cardiac ischemia. Two studies presented in abstract form measured some increases in power output during cycling exercise, but results were not statistically significant.

Ribose is for sale, so safety must be considered. Ribose has not been used for long periods of time, though doses of up to 20 grams appear to be tolerated. Higher doses may result in GI side effects. Manufacturer recommendations are often 3 grams prior to and 3 grams after exercise. The patent holder recommends that it be consumed with carbohydrates on an empty stomach. Current data is much too limited to safely recommend a cyclical or maintenance dose. In fact, much more data and solid proof is required before this supplement can be recommended.

Illegal Ergogenic Aids

Prohormone Products

Prohormones are widely sold in dietary supplements and are currently banned by the IOC and U.S. Antidoping. These products include the "andro" and "nor" prohormones. Andro products, namely androstenedione, are testosterone precursors, and transform to this hormone in the body. Other androgenic products include androstenediol and dehydroepiandrosterone (DHEA). Nor products are precursors to the steroid nortestosterone (nandrolone), which is similar in structure to testosterone. Available nor-prohormones are 19-norandrostenediol and 19-norandrostenedione. These nor products break down to the same metabolites used to detect nandrolone usage. Andro prohormones may lead to an elevated testosterone/epitestosterone ratio. All of these substances carry the risk of a positive drug test and potential negative side effects.

Since the late 1990s there has been a rash of elite athletes testing positive for the steroid nandrolone. Many of these athletes have claimed that it occurred through inadvertent ingestion of the dietary supplements that contained nor hormones. Prohormones are easily purchased in the U.S. and over the Internet because they are classified as dietary supplements. Often these supplements are geared toward muscle building, recovery, and "maintaining hormone levels."

While athletes can read labels carefully to avoid these banned products, it is becoming clear that this may not be enough. A study conducted at the UCLA

Olympic Laboratory checked urine tests after supplementation with androstene-dione and 19-norandrostenedione. As expected the 19-nor produced nandrolone metabolites exceeding IOC limits. But the results of the andro supplementation were especially concerning. This test actually produced nandrolone metabolites in the urine! Twenty of twenty-four positive urine samples exceeded IOC limits. Based on these findings, researchers tested several andro supplements. Seven of eight tested capsules contained varying amounts of 19-nor. Researchers speculated that the supplements had been contaminated with 19-nor in the manufacturing process. Many supplement companies use the same equipment to blend, encapsulate, and bottle both prohormone and non-prohormone products. Quality control is entrusted to supplement companies. It is estimated that only 30 percent of supplement companies actually achieve the standards met by pharmaceutical companies.

Some of these prohormones may carry some unwanted side effects (other than inadvertently testing positive). One study that supplemented with andro did not find higher testosterone levels or increased muscle strength, but actually an increase in blood estrogen and reduction in the good HDL cholesterol in male subjects. These side effects could result in potentially serious health effects. A second study tested andro combined with an herbal product designed to decrease estrogen production. The estrogenic profile was not reduced from the herbal supplements despite claims from the manufacturer.

Of course you should not take prohormones, because they are illegal. But read labels carefully to ensure that they are not inadvertently consumed in any products that you purchase, and be aware that cross contamination is a real concern. It may be prudent to purchase supplements from companies that do not also make prohormones.

Weight Loss Supplements

More than 17 million Americans purchased weight loss supplements from 1996 to 1998. Weight loss supplements are surrounded by strong claims and are often purported to speed up metabolism, burn fat, and decrease appetite. While several ingredients found in weight loss supplements are legal (and ineffective), some weight supplements are banned substances and may be dangerous to use.

The most widely purchased weight loss supplement is ephedra. It is also the supplement with the highest incidence of reported side effects. Ephedra or ephedrine or Ma Huang stimulates the central nervous system and improves appetite control. However, because of its stimulant nature, reported side effects include nervousness, headache, heart palpitations, dizziness, insomnia, and anxiety. Ephedra is also a banned substance, and its use will result in a positive test.

Overall, several hundred incidences of consumer illness and dozens of deaths have been reported with use of this product. The FDA has recommended that the amount of ephedra be limited in products and that labeling limit the recommended doses and provide adequate warning to consumers. While supplement companies contend that this product is safe in the recommended doses, many health care professionals do not consider this product safe. Individuals with hypertension or heart conditions and pregnant women absolutely should not use it. Because of the marketability of mixing weight loss ingredients, ephedra is often sold in combination with caffeine. This stimulant combination serves to exacerbate ephedra's potency and side effects. Health Canada recalled products containing more than 8 milligrams of ephedra per dose and those that combine ephedra and caffeine.

Another banned weight loss supplement with serious safety concerns is phenylpropanolamine (PPA), also known as norephedrine. This product claims to suppress appetite and stimulate metabolism. However, it can also increase the risk of bleeding stroke and its safety risks far outweigh its effectiveness. The FDA has warned consumers to stop immediate use of a product that contains PPA. In addition to PPA, this dietary weight loss supplement also contains caffeine, another herb called yohimbine, and diiodothyronine, a form of thyroid hormone. The FDA received multiple reports of livery injury or liver failure with use of this product over a two-week to three-month period.

You should exercise great caution in taking weight loss supplements. They can have negative health effects ranging from mild to serious and may contain banned products.

There are numerous ergogenic aids currently marketed to the endurance athlete. Unlike sports nutrition supplements such as sports drinks, recovery drinks, and gels, the claims behind most nutritional ergogenic aids remain scientifically unsupported. Creatine can benefit certain types of exercise that are not always relevant to an endurance athlete. Caffeine may also benefit some athletes but should be used carefully and within legal guidelines. Bicarbonate, while supported by research as an ergogenic aid, is unlikely to be of any benefit to endurance athletes.

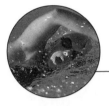

part **III**

SPORT SPECIFIC
NUTRITION GUIDELINES

How to Eat for Your Sport

Every endurance sport has unique nutritional considerations. While Parts I and II covered sports guidelines pertinent to all endurance athletes, Part III will focus on guidelines more specific to your sport. For example, the chapter on triathlon will address meal planning for multiple workouts and eating during an Ironman. Nutrition cycling considerations for competing in a road race, mountain bike race, and cyclo-cross race are covered in the cycling chapter.

Special nutrition considerations that pertain to endurance athletes in several sports are also covered in various chapters. Issues about training and racing in the heat will be covered in the cycling chapter. Nutritional strategies to prevent muscle cramping are covered in the triathlon chapter, while strategies for coping with cold weather are reviewed in the cross-country skiing chapter. You can cross-reference these topics as needed for your own personal training program and endurance sport focus.

191

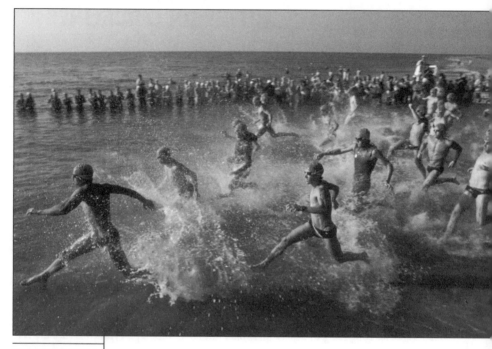

TOM MORAN PHOTO

chapter 9

NUTRITION FOR TRIATHLON

Triathlon is a popular and growing sport that made its Olympic debut in Sydney, Australia, at the 2000 Olympic Games. This multisport event includes professional and both serious elite and recreational age-group athletes. Triathlon race courses cover several distances. Often, triathletes train for only one distance, particularly Ironman competitions, while some triathletes may compete in one to two distances. Triathlon races are categorized according to the following distances:

Sprint distance: 0.5-mile swim, 12-mile cycle, and 3.1-mile run

Olympic distance: 0.93-mile swim, 24.8-mile cycle, and 6.2-mile run

Half Ironman: 1.2-mile swim, 56-mile cycle, and 13.1-mile run

Ironman: 2.4-mile swim, 112-mile cycle, and 26.2-mile run

Because they train for three distinct sports, triathletes have a busy schedule. Even age-group triathletes competing in a sprint distance race may train up to eight hours weekly. Triathletes competing in longer distances can spend anywhere from ten to thirty hours on weekly training. All triathletes have multiple training sessions, usually two daily. Training sessions may consist of aerobic training, interval training, weight training, and transition training. Triathletes often train year-round and may compete several times during the racing season, usually from late spring to early fall.

Depending on the level of the competitor, racing can last forty-five minutes for a sprint distance, four hours for Olympic distance, and up to a cut-off time of seventeen hours for the Ironman. While all race distances require specific nutritional preparation, the longer distances clearly present a serious nutritional challenge. Despite spreading the work out among various muscle groups used for swimming, cycling, and running, these longer distances will challenge your muscle fuel stores and blood glucose levels. Triathletes are also often challenged by the environmental conditions in which they complete a triathlon, which often take place in hot conditions that greatly increase the risk of dehydration and electrolyte depletion.

TRAINING NUTRITION CONCERNS

Timing Your Meals

As a triathlete, two-a-day training sessions may likely be a year-round part of your life. While these multiple training sessions are essential for refining your swimming, cycling, and running skills and accelerating conditioning, they also present a nutritional challenge. Your training places high energy demands upon your body and leaves limited hours for nutritional recovery between training sessions. It may seem sometimes that your life is one continuous cycle of training, eating, and recovery. That's probably because it is!

Determining how to time your meals and snacks around multisport training can be challenging. You don't want to train with an empty or even half-empty tank, or one that is too full prior to exercise. Figuring out just the right amount of fuel you need to train more than once daily can be tricky. Depending on when you have swimming, running, or cycling planned into your training schedule, you may find that eating several hours prior to exercise is uncomfortable.

Many triathletes find that their GI system can adapt fairly well to eating close to exercise, but clearly you must think ahead to the day's schedule in planning your food choices. Three factors will most likely affect your food choices—whether you are going for a swim, bike, or run, how hard you will train, and the timing of your training schedule. Generally the higher the intensity, the lighter the pre-exercise meal. Running will also likely present the greatest digestive challenge, with swimming next in line and cycling the most gentle on your GI system. While large meals before exercise could clearly make you drowsy and lethargic and possibly cause digestive distress, your real challenge is in determining the correct-size meal and meal choices that are optimal for you prior to a specific time and type of exercise session.

For the most part, a moderate-size snack providing one gram of carbohydrate per pound of weight can be consumed two hours prior to training. This snack can include some easily digested solid food, such as a granola bar and yogurt, along with fluids. If you need to eat within an hour of exercise, try an easily digested energy bar, piece of fruit, gel, or even 24 ounces of a sports drink to boost energy levels. It is important that you look ahead to your training schedule for that day. Perhaps your recovery foods will be a full meal, as this is what is most convenient for that day's program. Plan ahead and know when meals and snacks should be consumed so that you have the energy to train.

Early Morning Sessions

Early morning training sessions are not uncommon for the serious triathlete. Often this early session may be a swim, but could easily consist of a run or bike ride. If your early morning schedule does not leave much time for digestion, make sure that you consume a dinner, or perhaps even an evening snack, high in carbohydrates the night before. You want to start the training session with full muscle glycogen stores and minimize the effects of liver glycogen breakdown overnight as much as possible. You can also experiment with small, low-fiber snacks beforehand to determine tolerances. Some well-tolerated early morning noshes may include an energy bar, half a bagel or English muffin, small yogurt, glass of juice, or piece of fruit. These carbohydrate choices can keep your early morning blood glucose levels nice and steady. Aim for about 50–75 grams of carbohydrates before exercise. Of course, you should also drink plenty of water in the morning. If your early morning training session is a longer workout, you may also want to consider consuming a sports drink while you train. This strategy is easy on your GI system and ensures a steady supply of blood glucose. It can also compensate for eating a smaller amount of food before exercise.

During Training

Any time that your schedule or personal food tolerances preclude adequate food intake prior to training, think about what you can consume while exercising. Sports drinks, bars, and gels provide glucose for your exercising muscles and can offset muscle glycogen losses that occur later during exercise. Proper refueling during exercise prevents your body from entering a greatly depleted state and will ultimately speed your recovery. Try to consume 30–75 grams of carbohydrate per hour for workouts lasting longer than seventy-five minutes and during high intensity interval sessions. Consuming carbohydrates during training sessions is especially important if another training session will quickly follow with limited recovery time. Consecutive training sessions such as these occur during transition training.

Recovery Nutrition

Because you are in a constant cycle of training and recovery, it is very important that you pay close attention to recovery nutrition. If you go into your second workout dehydrated or low on energy, you may not have a high quality training session. In fact, you may end up digging yourself into an even bigger hole of energy depletion that will affect your training for the next day. Improper refueling can start a downward spiral of poor training and low energy. Follow the recovery nutrition guidelines in Chapter 4. Make sure that you plan to have foods on hand that will provide anywhere from 50 to 100 grams of carbohydrates and up to 20 grams of protein. Drink plenty of fluids and eat foods containing sodium after training in hot, humid weather.

What food choices would suit you best after exercise probably depends upon your training schedule. If your next training session is within two hours, a between-training-session snack is likely your best option. Aim for easily digested choices. One top age grouper enjoys a banana smoothie and toast with jam after a hard session, and knows that these foods will sit well until the next training session. Another may find that a recovery drink that can be mixed quickly after training or ahead of time is the most convenient choice. However, if your next training session is several hours away, you should consider having an actual meal. This will allow you to fill up not only on carbohydrates, but provide you with the opportunity to round out your protein and fat intake. Some triathletes practice both nutrition strategies after an arduous training block. They make certain that a good recovery snack is readily available immediately after training and follow this snack shortly afterward with a well-balanced meal.

FOOD AND YOUR TRAINING SCHEDULE

Clearly as a triathlete you need to plan ahead to have the proper meals and snacks available. Pack recovery foods and sports drinks the night before. Know what deli carries your favorite healthy lunch that provides just the right balance of protein, carbohydrate, and fat. And make sure that you have just the right afternoon snack available when hunger strikes or to prevent hunger during an early evening workout. The meal outline below reflects the food and training schedule of a half-Ironman competitor.

6:00 a.m.	8 ounces light yogurt, water, and juice
7:00 a.m.	45-minute easy run
8:30 a.m.	Cinnamon raisin bagel, peanut butter, fruit spread, and coffee
12:00 p.m.	Turkey sandwich topped with vegetables, pretzels, yogurt, and water
4:00 p.m.	Low fat granola, banana, milk, and water
5:30 p.m.	90-minute bike ride
8:00 p.m.	Broiled fish, rice, vegetables, bread, and water

If you train both in the morning and over the lunch hour, timing will be a bit tighter. After a strenuous morning workout, have recovery foods available in the form of a quick snack, followed by a large breakfast. If it is feasible, your recovery meal can be a nice-size breakfast. You may want to follow with a mid-morning snack so that hunger does not set in during your lunchtime training session. If needed, consume a sports drink during the lunchtime training session. Lunch should follow as your recovery meal. Depending on the intensity of your training, you may be hungry for an afternoon snack or an early dinner. The meals and snacks following your last training session of the day are your opportunity to refuel for the next day. Make sure that you continue to recover for the next twelve to twenty-four hours or up until the time when your next training session presents itself.

Evening training could definitely receive a good fuel boost from an afternoon snack. Later training sessions often take place five hours or more after your last good meal. Dinner can follow an evening training session as a recovery meal, and depending on the intensity of your training, you may even be hungry for an evening snack.

Energy and Weight

Optimal daily recovery refuels your body so that you can continue to train and reach your best potential. Don't underestimate your energy needs for triathlon training. Refer to the guidelines in Chapter 4 regarding energy requirements. Triathletes training for a sprint distance race clearly have lower energy requirements than an Ironman competitor whose energy needs may exceed 6,000 calories some days. But regardless of your competition focus, meeting your energy needs is essential for recovery. Attempts to lose weight quickly may be met with fatigue and lack-luster training. Keep in mind that optimum body fat levels are individual—an "ideal" weight that results in hormonal imbalance, loss of muscle and power, and compromised immune function will not make you a better triathlete. Lean triathletes who are also successful competitors achieve their low body fat levels through an intense training program. If you are interested in losing weight sensibly, refer to the weight management guidelines provided in Chapter 7.

COMPETITION NUTRITION CONCERNS

While you should start any triathlon well hydrated and well fueled, the distance in which you compete will determine your nutrition strategies for the week leading up to the race and during the race itself.

Sprint Triathlon

This shorter race still requires that you arrive at the start line with some previous nutritional planning and the proper training program. Focus on a diet ample in carbohydrates twenty-four to forty-eight hours prior to the race and have your energy needs match your training taper. Drink plenty of fluids to hydrate well and have a good high carbohydrate dinner the night before the race. Time your pre-race meal on race morning according to your personal preferences and tolerances, with plenty of fluids and easily digested foods. Drink fluids liberally before race time and time bathroom breaks appropriately to avoid becoming dehydrated during your warm-up prior to the race.

Enjoy the swim, have a good transition, and consume a sports drink on the bike leg of the competition. With typical race times ranging from just less than an hour to just less than two hours, it will be important for some sprint-distance triathletes to play it right nutritionally on the bike. Cycling presents the opportune time to drink and maintain blood glucose levels. By race day you should be a pro at on-bike drinking due to plenty of practice. Drink as you are able or desire for the quick run to the finish.

Olympic Distance

While top competitors may complete this race around the two-hour mark, for many age groupers an Olympic distance triathlon is a test of both technique and endurance, with four-hour finishes commonly listed in race results.

9.1

COMPETITION NUTRITION FOR SPRINT AND OLYMPIC DISTANCE TRIATHLON

Sprint Distance

Taper and consume adequate carbohydrates 24 hours before the race

Hydrate continually 48 hours before the race

Consume a high carbohydrate pre-race meal 2–3 hours prior to start time

Consume fluids from a sports drink leading up to the race

Drink 20–32 ounces of fluid every hour on the bike

Keep up with fluid needs as much as possible during the run

Olympic Distance

Taper and consume adequate carbohydrates 48 hours prior to the race

Hydrate continuously 48 hours prior to the race

Consume a high carbohydrate pre-race meal providing 1 g of carbohydrate per pound of weight 2–3 hours before start time

Increase salt intake 48 hours prior to the race if it will take place in hot and humid conditions

Consume fluids such as sports drinks in the hours leading up to the race

Consume 20–32 ounces of fluid every hour on the bike and consume carbohydrate gels with water if desired

Stop at aid stations for water to maintain fluid intake and minimize fluid losses

Again, eat according to your energy needs as determined by your taper for twenty-four to forty-eight hours and emphasize high carbohydrate foods. Try to time and size your meals appropriately for your start time, consuming 1.5–2.0 grams of carbohydrates per pound of weight three to four hours prior to the race (see Table 5.4). You may wish to time your pre-race meal closer to the start time and should decrease your carbohydrate intake accordingly. Practice the pre-race fluid tips outlined in Chapter 5 so that you start the race well hydrated. When you complete the swim and start the bike, begin fueling up with a sports drink. Some competitors may also prefer gels and water for their carbohydrate and fluid combination. If you are going to race in hot and humid conditions, make sure that the sports nutrition products you use contain adequate amounts of sodium. You can also increase your regular sodium intake the two days before the race to prevent sodium depletion.

Often the age groupers who have longer finish times can place themselves at a greater risk of sodium depletion. Ingesting low sodium fluids such as water over several hours can dilute blood and reduce sodium to below normal levels.

You should still focus on maintaining an adequate fluid intake during the run. Chances are that your efforts on the bike have not replaced 100 percent of your fluid, carbohydrate, and electrolyte losses. Drinking during the run is not as easy as during cycling, but you can practice and acquire this technique in training.

Ironman Nutrition

Preparing for Competition

The impact of optimal nutrition when competing in an Ironman triathlon cannot be overestimated. Having a good fluid and food day can make or break your race. Ironman triathletes are often progressively searching for the perfect food and fluid choices, and many top competitors have developed their own distinct rehydration and refueling choices and strategies. Ironman competition is grueling, so it is imperative that you begin the race with glycogen-loaded muscles, adequate liver glycogen stores, optimal hydration and topped-up fluid levels, and a placid and satisfied gastrointestinal system. One recent study measured that male Ironman competitors burned more than 10,000 calories of fuel during the race, and female competitors more than 8,000 calories. Energy intakes, however, were less than half the amount of calories burned.

Eating for the Taper

Regular Ironman training can take up to thirty hours weekly and necessitates a high calorie intake comprised of the proper balance of carbohydrates, fats, and proteins. However, Ironman competitors also taper training prior to competition. This allows the body to be fully recovered before the race, and presents the opportunity to refuel and carbohydrate load. It is important to appreciate that you may actually taper your training by a full 50 percent below normal and that this reduction in training reduces your calorie and carbohydrate requirements.

Even though you may be carbohydrate loading the week or so before an Ironman, your calorie and carbohydrate requirements may actually dip below training levels. When you carbohydrate load, you rest your muscles and burn minimal amounts of glycogen. You then eat to exceed your carbohydrate requirements in order to bring your glycogen levels to above normal. Your typical training diet should be more than adequate to accomplish this pre-race loading. In fact, continuing your normal caloric intake can lead to unwanted weight gain as you may only be training one to two hours daily.

During the carbohydrate loading phase of your program, your portions may be smaller than on training days. But do maintain a high percentage of your calories from carbohydrates. Of course, it is the total grams of carbohydrates that matter most, rather than percentages. If you are training up to two hours daily, consume anywhere from 3.0–4.5 grams of carbohydrates for every pound that you weigh. For a 165-pound triathlete this requires a carbohydrate intake of at least 500 grams daily, a significant amount that still requires knowledge and planning, though not as challenging as consuming 700 grams daily. Gauge your hunger and fullness carefully. If you are too hungry or become hungry quickly, you are not eating enough to fuel up your body. However, feelings of uncomfortable fullness are not appropriate either.

At the very least, your normal diet will fill up your muscle glycogen stores during a taper; at worst you will gain some weight. But do keep in mind that a bit of weight gain may be inevitable, as the glycogen you store in your body will hold water in your muscles. This fluid gain does not have detrimental effects upon your performance and provides precious fluid during competition.

Carbohydrates clearly matter the week prior to competition, but another important focus of your pre-race nutrition should be staying optimally hydrated. Fluid intake is especially important when you are racing where heat and humidity can reach an extreme level. Your daily fluid requirements regardless of training are several quarts daily. During training, average sweat rate losses can range from 1 to 3 quarts per hour. If possible, weigh yourself before and after training during your taper phase and consume 24 ounces of hydrating fluid for every pound of weight lost. A large volume of clear urine should be an adequate indicator of hydration. Pay close attention to your sodium requirements during this time as well. Have recovery drinks containing sodium, and add sodium to the foods you eat for several hours after training.

Chances are you will be traveling locally, nationally, or perhaps even internationally to compete in an Ironman. Pack some of your favorite foods such as sports nutrition supplements and portable items such as cereals, dried fruit, and granola bars. You can also call ahead to your destination and surf the Internet to determine what types of restaurants and menus are offered near where you are staying.

Even though well-trained triathletes are already glycogen storage machines, the forty-eight hours before a race is a critical time for true carbohydrate loading and ensuring optimal fuel stores. While you may simply eat "normally" during your taper, you can increase your carbohydrate intake two days before the race. Aim for 4–5 grams of carbohydrates per pound of weight. Forty-eight hours prior to racing, the types of carbohydrates you choose are just as important as the amounts you consume. Placing less emphasis on higher fiber foods can keep your gastrointestinal system settled and help you "race light." You should try to rely on carbohydrate-containing fluids and lower fiber foods. Concentrated low fiber carbohydrate sources also include jam, honey, soft drinks, energy bars, refined pastas, breads, cereals, sports drinks, and concentrated sports nutrition supplements. During this 48-hour period, you may need to streamline your protein and fat intake to make room for the carbohydrates.

You also don't want to encounter any digestive surprises in the forty-eight hours prior to Ironman competition. Make sure to limit hard-to-digest foods, excess fat and spices, and any unusual or new items. Stick with bland, simple, plain foods, and request special preparation as needed. Your meals may not be a culinary delight two days prior to racing, but at least they won't talk back to you during the race.

Many Ironman competitors have become very sodium conscious in recent years due to increasing and often visible cases of hyponatremia or low sodium blood levels that occur during the race. Certain individuals may be more susceptible to excess sodium losses than others, and what you consume before an Ironman can also make a difference. Some pre-race options include consuming high sodium foods and salting your food at light to heavy levels. Levels of sodium sweat losses and regulation of blood sodium levels are unique to each individual, but it would be prudent to start an Ironman with sodium blood levels at the high end of normal. Fluid intake also remains crucial two days before a race. Drink continuously during this pre-race period.

The Night Before

The night before an Ironman, easily digested, tried and true favorite foods low in fiber are your best option. Many athletes like potatoes, rice, refined breads, and pasta choices with a mild sauce, and also limit salads and other raw vegetables. You can also have a reasonable amount of easily digested protein with the night-before meal. A late evening snack can also provide a little carbohydrate insurance.

Race Morning

Race morning is another time where you will make important pre-race decisions regarding your food and fluid intake. Breakfast is a time to refill your liver glycogen stores after the overnight fast that occurs when you sleep, to top off your fluid levels to carry you through the swim and through T1, and to allow you to get settled on the bike. Small amounts of easily digested protein can also work for some competitors the morning of the race. Experiment with some of your favorite choices in training, and don't try anything new on race day. Table 9.2 summarizes some Ironman pre-race nutrition strategies.

During the Race

Despite all your heroic efforts to prepare nutritionally prior to an Ironman, consuming adequate calories and carbohydrate during an Ironman is essential to completing the race and performing your best. Optimal eating and drinking fuels you

IRONMAN PRE-RACE NUTRITION STRATEGIES

THE WEEK BEFORE THE RACE

Timing	Nutrition Strategies
2–7 days prior to competition	■ Consume your regular training diet or decrease portions slightly to compensate for training taper ■ Maintain at least 3 grams carbohydrates per pound of weight ■ Adequate intake of fluids ■ Increase intake of salt and salty foods
48 hours prior to competition	■ Load with 4–5 grams of carbohydrates per pound weight ■ Emphasize low-fiber foods and carbohydrates containing fluids ■ Consume adequate amounts fluid and sodium
Night before	■ Emphasize low fiber carbohydrates ■ Consume easily digested protein as desired ■ Avoid high fiber foods ■ Consume an evening snack if desired ■ Drink plenty of fluids
Morning of the race	■ 2–3 hours prior consume 1 g carbohydrates per pound weight ■ Have easily digested carbohydrates ■ Consume carbohydrate-electrolyte beverage for carbohydrates and fluids

SODIUM CONTENT OF FOODS

Salt, 1 tsp.	2,300 mg
Canned soup, 1 cup	900–1,400 mg
Pretzels, 1 oz.	451 mg
Luncheon meats, 1 oz.	200–500 mg
Crackers, 1 oz.	100–400 mg
Salted nuts, 1 oz.	100–200 mg

SAMPLE PRE-RACE MEALS

High carbohydrate sports supplement Energy bar	Soy milk, 16 oz. Cereal, low fiber, 1 1/2 cups High-carbohydrate sports supplement
English muffins, 2 Jam, 2 Tbsp. Sports drink, 24 oz.	Oatmeal, cooked, 1 cup Toast, 2 slices Spread, 1 tsp., and Jam, 2 Tbsp. Sports drink, 32 oz.

to the finish after months of preparation, whereas inadequate nutritional intake can leave you feeling depleted and disappointed. When preparing for your Ironman competition, it certainly can't hurt to visualize a "good stomach day."

As an Ironman competitor you need to translate the nutrition guidelines for eating and drinking during exercise into combinations and amounts of sports drinks, sodium sources, gels, bars, and other foods that work for your individual preferences and tolerances and maintain your energy levels toward the finish.

As in your pre-race preparation, the most important nutrients during racing remain fluid, carbohydrates, and sodium. In order to maintain an adequate fluid intake you have to appreciate that sweat rates can range from 1 to 3 quarts per hour. These fluid losses vary with heat, humidity, exercise intensity, acclimatization, and fitness levels. The more pronounced the factors, the greater your fluid losses. You should also appreciate that studies indicate that fluid empties from your stomach with much individual variability, but generally at rates of 24 to 40 ounces per hour. Aim to consume this amount of fluid and practice in training.

Sodium remains an important nutrient during an Ironman. Estimated sodium losses from sweating range from 115 to 700 milligrams per hour, but can be as high as 2,000 milligrams per hour in non-acclimated athletes. You can obtain sodium from sports drinks. Check labels of your favorite products to determine their sodium content. You can also add small amounts of salt to a sports drink if needed. One-quarter of a teaspoon of salt contains 550 milligrams of sodium. Salt tablets generally contain several hundred milligrams of sodium per tablet. All salt tablets should be consumed with at least 8 ounces of water.

Of course, you need carbohydrates to maintain blood glucose levels and provide fuel for your muscles as glycogen stores are burned for energy. Try to replace carbohydrates at a rate of 0.5 grams or 2 calories per pound of weight per hour. This translates to about 60–100 grams of carbohydrates or 250–400 calories per hour, as Ironman competitors expend several thousand calories in a race. Generally 32 ounces of a sports drink provides 55–75 grams of carbohydrates. Check labels of any items such as energy bars or gels that you may consume during a race for their carbohydrate content.

T1 and On-the-Bike Nutrition

After a swim in choppy waters or salt water, your stomach may feel a bit unsettled. You may swallow some water during the swim and even feel a bit nauseous. But the bike leg is your opportunity to consume adequate fuel and set yourself up for the run. It is also the longest leg of the triathlon. Try not to wait more than thirty minutes before you start consuming fluids.

Once you and your stomach are settled on the bike leg, it is time to get down to business. Start consuming fluids as soon as you can tolerate them. Fuller stomachs empty faster and quickly replace sweat losses. Sports drinks can provide a perfect balance of fluid and carbohydrates and varying amounts of sodium. Plain water can wash down the taste of sweet gels and beverages in hot and humid conditions.

Try out your favorite sports drink and gels (and the brand on the race course) during longer bike rides that are near race pace. The more efficient you become at drinking on the bike, the less energy you expend. You may want to slow down slightly when you refuel, but the more you can maintain your pace, the better.

Despite the fact that biking keeps your stomach and GI system relatively stable, most triathletes prefer to consume the majority of their calories from fluids. Gels are also well tolerated. Many top competitors have also come up with their own fluid replacement formula, often having something a bit more concentrated than a sports drink, and perhaps even adding a bit of protein and salt as well. Of course, anyone who consumes these personalized products has experimented with them in training. As far as solids are concerned, they are generally kept to a minimum but can provide a nice chew in the middle of all that drinking. Make sure that you limit solids to well-proven, tolerable foods. Some possible options are fruit bars, cut-up sports bars, and bananas. But only your stomach knows for sure what works best. You can also take along some items that you may possibly crave.

Muscle Cramps

If you have ever suffered a muscle cramp, you probably remember how it felt. These sustained muscle spasms can be painful and inconvenient, particularly when they occur during competition. While the exact cause of muscle cramps largely remains a mystery, they are generally associated with longer exercise sessions in the heat and overexertion. However, there are some basic nutritional steps that you can take to possibly prevent muscle cramps.

Research suggests that muscle cramps are related to salt imbalances. Muscle cramps during exercise have been linked to either large losses of sodium chloride in sweat, to replacing sweat losses with dilute fluid low in sodium, or a combination of the two. Dehydration and mineral deficiencies may also be predisposing factors. One age grouper experienced severe muscle cramps during her first long-distance triathlon, though never in training. She increased her salt intake when training in hot, humid weather and prior to her next competition. Fortunately, she no longer suffered from muscle cramping by employing this strategy.

It is important to maintain adequate hydration levels before, during, and after exercise. Consume at least 8 ounces of fluid every hour. Monitor urine color and volume. Your urine should be pale to clear if you are well hydrated. During exercise try to consume up to 8 ounces of fluid every fifteen to twenty minutes. Check your weight before and after exercise. Rehydrate by consuming 24 ounces of fluid for every pound of weight lost during exercise. You should also be able to urinate shortly after prolonged exercise if you are adequately rehydrated.

It would also be prudent to obtain plenty of sodium in your diet while training in hot weather and becoming acclimatized. Guidelines for restricting sodium are often appropriate for individuals with high blood pressure, but may not be appropriate for many endurance athletes. Foods that contain sodium include canned soups, pretzels, cereals, cheese, crackers, and yogurt. You can also salt your food prior to hot training or competition days. If you find yourself craving salt, your body may be telling you that it requires more sodium.

It has also been speculated that potassium losses can lead to muscle cramping, though sodium losses are the most likely culprit. Your diet can easily supply ample amounts of potassium. Excellent sources include fruit juices, fruit, vegetables, milk, yogurt, and dried peas and beans. You may want to eat generous portions of these foods anyway, as they provide carbohydrates.

A lack of calcium is often blamed for muscle cramps, though this has not been conclusively proven. Calcium is the most abundant mineral in your body and plays many functional roles, including muscle contraction. However, it is not highly likely that your blood levels will fall below normal, as the huge calcium stores in your bones will supply calcium as needed. But making sure to consume enough calcium won't hurt and will help preserve bone mass. Good sources of calcium, which include milk, yogurt, and leafy green vegetables, are listed in Chapter 3. A calcium supplement can also compensate for a low dietary intake of this important mineral. Another theory is that a lack of magnesium, a mineral that plays an important role in muscle relaxation, may be related to muscle cramping. Good sources of magnesium include nuts, seeds, legumes, green leafy vegetables, and unrefined grains.

Muscle cramps may not be solely related to nutritional issues. In fact, modifying training techniques and improved stretching may be the solutions to your muscle cramps if other strategies fall short. ■

Pack more gels, bars, and other treats than you think you will need. This allows you to have some choices and satisfy cravings. You can tape gel packets to your bike for easy handling or plant them ahead of time in a pack or the pockets of a cycling jersey. Experiment with various carrying systems. You may want to try a bladder hydration system or seat mounted and aerobar mounted bottle carriers in addition to the traditional mounted water bottles. Pack your turnaround bag with fluids and foods and allow yourself some choices so that you can pick the item that is most appealing at that time.

Practice keeping up with your fluid requirements. Once you become dehydrated it can become difficult to empty fluids adequately from your stomach. As you attempt to catch-up with your fluid losses and drink more, your stomach will become uncomfortable and bloated. Despite your intake of fluids, you may experience the symptoms of fluid and carbohydrate depletion. It can be hard to differentiate between the symptoms of requiring more fluid or more carbohydrate. If you don't need to urinate, then you are not emptying adequately.

T2 and the Run

Maintaining proper hydration and carbohydrate intake is challenging on the run. Running is harder on your GI system than cycling and more likely to result in nausea and bloating. By the time the running leg rolls around, you have been exercising for several hours and only partially replaced your fluid losses. You may feel fluid jostling around in your stomach. It is important that you stop or slow down at aid stations and make a point to drink fluids as much as possible. Most competitors choose to stay away from solids and stick with water, sports drinks, gels, and cola during the run. Because the risks of hyponatremia can increase as the race progresses, many competitors also bring along salt tablets.

There are a variety of steps that you can employ to set yourself up for good GI tolerance during the run. Which step you choose depends upon your own individual tolerances. Some competitors find that it is best not to consume anything for the last 15–30 minutes on the bike and keep their intake very light for the first few miles into the run. Other competitors successfully down a whole bottle of sports drink in T2. Knowing how you will fare best during this transition takes practice and experimentation in training.

Alternating between gels, sports drinks, water, and cola can support you in meeting your carbohydrate and fluid needs during the run. Alternating cola with water can help dilute the higher carbohydrate concentration of the drink. The caffeine in the cola may also stimulate your central nervous system and improve your focus and concentration during the race. Slow down when you approach aid stations. By the time you gulp fluid from the cups provided, you may actually down only 2 ounces in volume.

If you do consume gels during the run, make sure that you take them with plenty of fluid. Also look for some flavor varieties from your drinks to relieve the taste boredom that can occur. Switching to a different drink for part of the run may be just the change you need. Keep in mind that some gels and cola are not as high in sodium as sports drinks. Often competitors make a point of consuming salt tablets during the run, as they have become somewhat depleted of sodium and are consuming low sodium fluids. Make sure that you do not take excessive amounts of salt tablets and that you have no medical contraindication to taking these tablets. Also consume salt tablets with plenty of fluid. Triathletes who arrive from cooler environments and have not had time to acclimatize are at greater risk for hyponatremia. Slower triathletes are also at risk for developing low blood sodium levels. Longer race times provide more opportunity for sodium losses that are not adequately replaced with enough sodium-containing drinks and for a high fluid consumption.

Unfortunately it can be difficult to discern if your stomach is not emptying properly. Once you become dehydrated, your risk of GI upset increases significantly. Dehydration will delay fluids emptying from your stomach, and attempts to rehydrate will upset your stomach further. It is best not to stop drinking altogether. But if you do overfill and vomit, regroup and start drinking fluids again slowly.

The symptoms of not consuming enough carbohydrates, or not emptying fluids quickly and not absorbing enough carbohydrates, can be confusing. If you don't produce adequate amounts of urine, chances are that you are not emptying fluids quickly enough from your stomach.

Feeling mentally sharp can indicate that adequate glucose is available to fuel your brain. Feeling irritable or spacey may reflect low blood glucose levels. If symptoms of hypoglycemia occur, try a gel or soda and see if symptoms improve. Experienced triathletes appreciate that every Ironman is different and that a key to success is learning how to listen to your body and providing what it needs during the race.

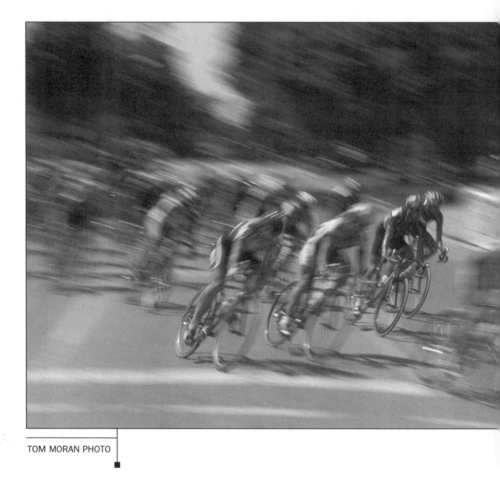

TOM MORAN PHOTO

chapter 10

NUTRITION FOR ROAD CYCLING, MOUNTAIN BIKING, AND CYCLO-CROSS

Cycling is undoubtedly one of the most challenging endurance sports. It requires muscular strength, power, and endurance for successful competition. Cyclists complete long aerobic training rides to prepare for competition, but also incorporate a significant amount of anaerobic exercise into a program that includes intervals, sprints, and weight training. It is important that cyclists develop both the aerobic and anaerobic systems in order to compete at their best.

Cyclists can compete in a number of events during the spring to fall season including road races that can vary in length from 15 to 80 miles, criterium racing, and time trialing. The sport of mountain biking is also popular, and in some areas of the country there is the opportunity to compete in track cycling. Cyclo-cross is also a traditional off-season option, and many cyclists may also choose to participate in strength training during this time of year.

Road racing requires muscular endurance, surges in speed, and the ability to sprint at the end of a race. Depending at which level you compete, road races may last from forty-five minutes to several hours. The extreme in road racing is exemplified by professional stage racing, particularly the twenty-one-day Tour de France. Mountain bike racing requires mainly muscular endurance, but also power for climbing steep hills and sprinting at the finish. Cyclo-cross is a shorter but very high intensity event that requires superb bike handling, the ability to handle varying terrain, and the skill of dismounting and mounting your bike. Track racing demands mostly power from the cyclist, though the training program will incorporate long endurance rides. Of course, many recreational riders also complete long bike rides and events in the warmer months, thus altering their nutritional requirements.

Cyclists typically train once daily but incorporate longer rides lasting several hours weekly, particularly on the weekends. Training will also include higher intensity rides or anaerobic threshold training, interval training, and sprint workouts. It is not unusual for cyclists to train between ten and twenty hours weekly.

TRAINING NUTRITION
Off-Season
During the off-season, cyclists concentrate on strength training and may train on the road or indoors on a wind trainer or rollers. Cyclists who live in parts of North America with friendly climates may put in some steady miles but overall complete less volume and intensity on the bike. You may also take a short break from cycling during this time and participate in other sports in order to crosstrain.

If you strength train, proper nutrition can make the most of your program. Strength training can help you maintain lean body mass that is normally lost with the aging process. It can also improve your aerobic performance and help prevent injury. Depending on your aerobic exercise, your overall calorie and carbohydrate requirements may be lower than during the height of the season when you are training more than fifteen hours weekly and completing training rides lasting several hours. As reviewed in Chapter 7, following specific nutrition guidelines optimizes weight training results.

You need to consume enough calories to build muscle. It takes 350–400 additional calories daily to build one pound of muscle. If you are trying to shed a few pounds during the off-season, strict dieting can hamper your muscle building efforts. Your protein intake should not increase significantly while weight training and may even be a bit lower than during the regular demanding training season, unless you are new to weight training. Protein requirements of 0.5 to 0.8 grams per pound of weight are easily met with a well-balanced diet and nutritious food choices.

Muscle glycogen is an important energy source during weight training, so arrive for training sessions in a well-fueled state. If your schedule does not allow for a pre-training snack, you can consider consuming a sports drink during training to maintain blood glucose levels, supply your muscles with fuel, and maintain adequate hydration. You should also practice recovery nutrition after a hard weight training session. Carbohydrates with or without a small amount of protein should be adequate to stimulate muscle glycogen resynthesis.

If you train outside during the colder months, you still need to replace fluid losses from sweating, though losses may not be as significant as in hot and humid weather. If you are dressed warmly, sweat losses can reach 2 liters per hour. Cold weather exercise can also cause fluid losses through exhalation as a result of a pressure gradient that is created between the cold air outdoors and the warm air in your lungs. Dehydration can increase your risk of frostbite by decreasing blood flow to the extremities. Keeping up with fluid losses is hard enough in warm weather and even more challenging in cold weather. Cold weather can also blunt your thirst, which in any case is not a sensitive indicator to stimulate drinking early enough.

During cold weather exercise, aim for consuming at least one full 20-ounce water bottle per hour. If the thought of a cold sports drink makes your teeth chatter, prepare your drink with warm or hot water. Hot decaffeinated tea mixed with plenty of honey can provide a carbohydrate boost. You can even dilute sweet drinks such as hot chocolate and hot apple cider for warming energy while training. These warm liquids provide several advantages. They are easier to drink when it is cold outside, provide a feeling of warmth, and increase blood flow to the extremities by dilating blood vessels. And better yet, your body does not need to expend the extra energy required to warm cold liquids. For the same reasons, keep any food you bring with you as warm as possible. Cold weather does create a greater demand for calories. Remain focused on carbohydrates, as shivering uses up this fuel source, and so do your muscles, even during longer, lower intensity "fat burning" rides. Eating closer to exercise can also have a warming effect. Make this meal or snack predominately carbohydrate.

Early Season

When warmer weather returns, or you are looking ahead to the upcoming racing calendar, the great outdoors may be beckoning for more miles, greater intensity, and even an early race or two. It is now time to carefully match what you burn on the bike with what you consume both on and off the bike. You may come into early season training a bit on the heavier side of your ideal racing weight and may be tempted to "diet" to shed a few pounds. Try to resist the temptation of reducing calories too severely and consuming no calories during longer rides. While these techniques may produce quick weight loss results, they can also produce negative results such as poor recovery, hypoglycemia during training, intense hunger and subsequent overeating, and can eventually hold you back in training. You don't want to end up feeling tired and overtrained just at the time when you were hoping to whip yourself into shape. After longer rides, you should also pay attention to the immediate post-exercise recovery nutrition guidelines outlined in Chapter 4.

Training and Racing Season

When training and racing season is in full gear, the amount of calories and carbo-hydrates your body expends becomes significant. Review Chapter 4 on daily recovery nutrition to ensure that you match your training with your carbohydrate intake and round out your meals with adequate protein and fat. It can be difficult for cyclists to meet their energy needs from three meals daily. Plan on having snacks and possibly even incorporating caloric sports nutrition supplements into your diet. For some cyclists, energy needs may exceed 4,000 to 6,000 calories on heavy training days, an impossible food consumption task without careful planning and plenty of meals and snacks. Most successful cyclists are constantly grazing during the day. Large meals may make you feel heavy and sleepy, while several steady meals and snacks keep the recovery process going throughout the day.

Recovery nutrition is essential after long training rides. You need 0.5 grams of carbohydrates per pound of body weight and smaller amounts of protein within thirty minutes after exercise to recover. When you train in hot and humid weather, make sure that you also consume some sodium afterward to replace electrolyte losses and optimize your hydration status. Have these recovery snacks readily available after rides. Fluids are also an important part of your daily training diet. Carry or have fluid with you everywhere you go, on public transportation, in the car, and at your desk. Keep drinking and make sure that you produce several full bladders of clear urine daily. Follow the daily hydration guidelines presented in Chapter 1. Check your weight before and after hard training. Consume 24 ounces of fluid for every pound lost. If you are losing greater than 1 to 2 pounds of fluid weight during training, you are not keeping up with your fluid requirements as closely as you should.

Cyclists should also pay close attention to their iron and calcium intake. They can lose large amounts of iron through sweating and may have elevated iron requirements from their heavy training. Female cyclists should be especially careful to include good iron sources in their diet because of higher iron losses, though male cyclists are susceptible to being deficient in this nutrient as well. Have a sports medicine physician monitor your iron stores, and supplement safely if necessary.

Cycling is not considered a weight-bearing sport, though it does put some pressure on your spine. However, cyclists need to pay close attention to maintaining good bone health and preventing osteoporosis—for both men and women. While osteoporosis is a multifactorial disease, consistent weight-bearing exercise and adequate calcium intake are two of the cornerstone recommendations for preventing this debilitating condition. Cyclists should incorporate weight-bearing exercise into their training year-round and consume at least 1,000 milligrams of calcium daily. If your diet does not provide this amount of calcium, a calcium supplement can make up the difference.

Body fat levels are also a big concern for cyclists. Many successful elite and professional competitors are extremely lean, but they also put in long hours of training, which is the most effective way to safely reach low levels of body fat. Severe dieting or attempts to become too lean can result in fatigue, loss of muscle mass and power, and possibly overtraining. Follow the guidelines for sensible weight loss presented in Chapter 7, and remember that a good cycling program requires quite a bit of energy to be successfully maintained. Be patient, and let the weight take care of itself with good training and proper eating.

FOOD AND FLUID DURING LONG RIDES

Cycling is a unique endurance sport in that refueling while you train is a relatively simple task. No other sport keeps your stomach and gastrointestinal system so stable or conveniently allows you to carry your food and fluids. This is fortunate as the fluid and carbohydrate demands during training are high. Cyclists experience significant fluid losses, though they may be unaware of this as their sweat evaporates quickly in the wind. This wind effect can also keep you from overheating and hide your need for fluid. Start training with a moderate volume of fluid to distend your stomach and to enhance emptying, and start drinking as soon as you settle into the rhythm of your training ride. Aim for 4 to 8 ounces every fifteen to twenty minutes. Set your watch or heart rate monitor to remind yourself to drink on schedule. Once you become dehydrated, it will be difficult to catch up with your fluid requirements. Remember that riding in the heat, wind, or humidity also increases your fluid losses and therefore your fluid requirements.

You will dip significantly into your muscle glycogen stores when endurance rides last longer than 1.5 hours, and during interval and sprint training lasting more than one hour. To obtain both fluid and carbohydrates, it makes sense that you consume a sports drink during these types of rides. Cyclists seem to be more susceptible than other endurance athletes to bonking, or low blood glucose levels. Consuming a sports drink will maintain blood glucose and provide your muscles with a fuel source when they run low on glycogen. If you anticipate a longer training ride, consume a sports drink from the start. You can also bring along gels, bars, or bananas if you need a change from liquid carbohydrates. Just as it is difficult to catch up with your fluid needs when you are already dehydrated, it can also be challenging to consume carbohydrates when your blood sugar is already low, so hypoglycemia is best prevented.

Because food and fluid can be carried on your bike, you can pack large water bottles filled with sports drink. For longer rides, pack powdered drinks and reconstitute them in your emptied bottles along the way. For larger volumes you can carry a bladder system. These bladder systems also work well during more technical off-road rides during which you may not wish to take your hands off the handlebars. You can also pack gels and bars in your jersey pockets or tuck them conveniently in the leg of your cycling shorts. If you find the taste of sports drinks too sweet in hot weather, look for milder or unflavored drinks. You can also alternate a swig of a sweet sports drink with a gulp of water.

Another technique for preparing yourself nutritionally is to eat and drink plenty of fluid before a long training ride. Start with a good breakfast two hours beforehand and consume plenty of carbohydrates according to the guidelines presented in Chapter 5. If you train in the evening, make sure to have a substantial afternoon snack providing 50–100 grams of carbohydrates one to two hours beforehand. Before very early morning rides, you may not have time for a good breakfast other than downing something simple such as juice and toast. Make sure you consume carbohydrates during the ride to offset low morning liver glycogen stores.

COMPETITION NUTRITION

What a cyclist eats in the days and hours before an important race can make a positive performance impact for races lasting more than sixty minutes. Smart pre-race eating provides several performance benefits. In particular, cyclists can lower their chances of developing hypoglycemia or low blood sugar or "bonking," along with the accompanying feelings of fatigue, poor concentration, and light-headedness. Eating right for the race can also "top off" your muscle glycogen stores and provides your exercising muscles with fuel during the race. Eating before racing will also settle your stomach and prevent hunger pains during longer races. Any fluids you consume in the pre-race meal and hyperhydrating before competition also decreases your risk of developing dehydration during the race. You will also benefit psychologically from knowing that your race-ready body has been properly fed.

Cyclists should arrive at any race lasting longer than sixty minutes with adequate body stores of carbohydrates. Depending on your racing schedule, rest or taper for twenty-four to forty-eight hours and consume a diet adequate in carbohydrates. You can load up on carbohydrates before longer criteriums, time trials, and road races. It is especially important to rest and replenish your stores before a series of races.

The foods you choose, the amounts you consume, and how you time your pre-race meal will largely be determined by your race start time, the type of race in which you are competing, and your personal tolerances. For races lasting longer than sixty minutes, consume 30 to 60 grams of carbohydrates per hour to prevent hypoglycemia and provide muscles with fuel later in exercise. However, consuming fluids during racing is not as simple as fluid consumption during training. Depending on the type of race, bike racing requires that you respond to sudden changes in speed, race tactics, and varying terrain.

Road Racing

Road race start times can be as early as 8:00 a.m. and as late as 4:00 p.m. for the various racing categories. You may also have to travel to the race and eat your pre-race meal in the early morning hours, on the road, or even in the car. For road races that last longer than one hour, you should rest and consume adequate carbohydrates for twenty-four to forty-eight hours. Most cyclists prefer to consume their pre-race meal two-and-a-half to three hours beforehand. As reviewed in Chapter 5, consume about one gram of carbohydrates per pound of weight, more if tolerated during this time.

Small amounts of low fat protein and tiny amounts of fat can also be included if your tolerances allow. Make sure to provide enough extra digestion time to compensate for pre-race nerves.

If you have an early start time, it may still be worth eating two hours prior to exercise and allowing time to warm up. You can make this meal especially high in easy-to-digest carbohydrates such as liquid carbohydrates and sports nutrition supplements. If you need to consume a smaller meal, consume ample amounts of a sports drink in the hour leading up to the race for both extra carbohydrates and hydration. Later morning starts may simply allow time for a large pre-race breakfast three or even four hours beforehand. You can top off this meal with an easily digested item an hour before exercise providing 50–75 grams of carbohydrates, and of course consume plenty of fluids. Late afternoon start times may allow you to sleep later and have a large pre-race breakfast followed by a snack. You can also consider having an early breakfast and a small lunch-type meal two hours prior to the start time. Experiment with various start times and meals in training. Try to mimic the start time scenario of the most important races of the season during training.

During road races you should make an effort to maintain good hydration levels early on. If the race lasts more than ninety minutes, a sports drink can maintain blood glucose levels and provide fuel for glycogen depleted muscles later in the race. Make sure to drink gulps when the pace is relatively steady, as surges in the race may preclude drinking on the bike at various times during the race. Large volumes of fluid leave your stomach more rapidly than sips, and there won't be the steady opportunity to drink as during training. Practice your drinking technique in training as much as possible, and follow the pre-hydration guidelines from Chapter 5, starting thirty-six to forty-eight hours before the race. Make sure that you drink adequately during your warm-up. Aim to drink two water bottles of fluid the morning of the race.

During longer road races you may wish to try more concentrated sources of carbohydrates such as gels and pieces of energy bars. Just make sure to consume them

Training and Racing in the Heat

As an endurance athlete, it is highly likely that you often train and race in hot and humid conditions. Physiologically, heat is the most severe stressor that you can encounter while training, as your body must cope with both the heat generated from exercise and the heat of the environment.

Training in the heat stresses your body through a number of physiological responses, and it is important that you appreciate that extreme heat limits your ability to train. When you train, your muscles rely on a sufficient blood supply that carries needed oxygen and fuel. Eventually, the heat produced in very hot weather can become so great that neither your muscles nor skin receive adequate blood flow to maintain exercise and sufficient body cooling.

In very hot training conditions, sweating is your body's primary mechanism for shedding excess heat and maintaining a safe body core temperature. To cool your body effectively through sweating, sweat must evaporate and not just drip off your skin. However, on very humid days the air is already saturated with water and consequently less sweat is evaporated. Your risk of becoming dehydrated and developing heat illness is even greater when you train in both heat and humidity.

Just as when training in cooler temperatures, you must replace the fluid lost through sweat or dehydration will result. You may sweat anywhere from 2 to 3 quarts of fluid per hour while training in the heat. Even losing as little as 2 percent of your body weight can impair your training efforts.

In addition to greater fluid losses and increased body temperature, training in the heat imposes other stresses on your body. When you train in hot weather, your body demands an increased rate of muscle glycogen use, which can result in premature fatigue. Lactic acid production is also greater and your heart rate increases to compensate for fluid losses. Consequently, training at a given intensity is harder.

The key to training in hot weather is to appreciate that your body must adapt to the heat. While a few training sessions of thirty to sixty minutes at 70 percent of VO_2 max may be helpful, full adaptation to the heat may take from seven to fourteen days and is a highly individual response. After ten days of training in the heat, the sweat response adapts in several ways—you start to sweat sooner, your sweat rate increases, there is a greater distribution of sweat over your body, and your sweat contains fewer electrolytes to lessen your sodium losses. Other

adaptations include an increased blood volume and decreased sodium excretion in the urine. After ten days of training in the heat, your sweating capacity during exercise can double.

While these adaptations are all essential to cooling your body, they do result in greater fluid losses. Clearly, if these fluid losses are not replaced, you run the risk of becoming dehydrated and the benefits of heat acclimatization are lost. Because your sweat capacity is greatly enhanced after adapting to the heat, dehydration can occur quickly. And in addition to fluid replacement, you should also emphasize glucose replacement to meet the accelerated fuel demands imposed by training in the heat.

Start training well hydrated. Consume 16 ounces of fluid before bedtime, and in the early morning consume 16–24 ounces of fluid. Prior to training you should consume 8–10

(continued on page 226)

(continued from page 225)

ounces of fluid every hour. Then you can start to hyperhydrate one hour before exercise by consuming 16–32 ounces of fluid. Twenty minutes prior to training drink another 8–16 ounces. In the hour before exercise, a sports drink may be your best fluid choice. These drinks provide carbohydrates for fuel, and the sodium they contain can increase fluid retention. Try to start training with a nice volume of fluid in your stomach, as fluid empties more quickly when your stomach is stretched. Experiment to determine what volumes are in your comfort level.

Often, whether or not you can keep up with fluid losses is a matter of practicality. Consuming the amounts of fluid you require can be challenging due to logistics, limited opportunities to drink, availability of fluid, and practice. Aim to consume 4–8 ounces of fluid every fifteen to twenty minutes during exercise. Set your watch to remind you to drink at specific intervals. Take big gulps so fluids empty more quickly from your stomach. Start drinking right away. If you become dehydrated, fluid empties more slowly from your stomach.

When your training session lasts longer than ninety minutes, or sixty minutes at high intensity, your best fluid choice is likely to be a sports drink. The carbohydrates in the drinks offset muscle and liver glycogen losses, help maintain blood glucose levels, and supply your muscles with fuel later in exercise.

Sports drinks also provide the important electrolyte sodium. Sodium and chloride, which form salt, are the major electrolytes lost in sweat. When you go out for a very long training session or compete in races lasting several hours, you may be at risk for developing hyponatremia or low blood sodium levels. Hyponatremia results from losing large amounts of salt from sweating and replacing fluid losses with plain water. Essentially you dilute the sodium concentration in your blood.

To prepare for these sodium losses, you can increase your intake of salty foods or salt the day or two before a long ride or race, unless this is medically contraindicated. Avoid drinking plain water when a sports drink or sodium-containing gel plus water can be consumed to maintain blood sodium levels. If plain water tastes better in the heat, consider one of the sports drinks with little or no flavor. These products are often very appealing in hot weather. The sodium found in sports drinks improves their taste and can also enhance fluid and glucose absorption through the small intestine, and may enhance the thirst and drinking mechanism.

Both rehydration and refueling are also top priorities after exercising in the heat. You want to fully restore fluid losses from one training session to the next and bear in mind that thirst is not a reliable indicator of fluid losses. When you are thirsty, you are already dehydrated. The thirst mechanism also shuts down before you have sufficiently replaced all your fluid losses.

Weigh yourself before and after training. Try to consume 24 ounces of fluid for every pound of weight lost to replace both sweat and subsequent urine losses. Sweeter products or something a bit salty may stimulate your desire to drink. Cool drinks are usually more palatable.

Sodium or salt may stimulate your drive to drink, and also enhance the rehydration process. Sweating results in large fluid losses and relatively small sodium losses. After training, your blood volume and total body water are reduced, while there is a mild increase in blood

(continued on page 228)

(continued from page 227) concentration and sodium content. Consuming large amounts of plain water after exercise can dilute your blood before your full blood volume has been restored. This dilution effect shuts down the thirst mechanism, and you urinate to bring your blood con- centration back to normal. The end result is that you will produce a large amount of dilute urine before you are fully rehydrated. You can prevent this from occurring by including sodium in your recovery drinks, but also empha- size salty foods after exercise to replenish fluid stores properly. ■

with at least 6–8 ounces of fluid. If you are racing in very hot weather, sports drinks are probably your best choice. You can also alternate one bottle of a sports drink with water in hot weather racing. Some very disciplined elite racers can consume one full bottle every half-hour. Practice will also improve your ability to drink at very high intensities. Aim for 30–60 grams of carbohydrates hourly from the various products you consume and tolerate while racing. Commit to a specific number of bottles for the entire race, and try to drink on schedule. Practice your technique for receiving additional food and fluid in the feed zone.

If you are competing over the weekend in several back-to-back daily races, make sure that you pay close attention to recovery nutrition. Pack supplemental products to ensure that you meet your carbohydrate needs and replenish glycogen stores prior to the next start time. When eating at restaurants, emphasize concentrated car- bohydrate sources such as pasta, rice, potatoes, breads, and cereals. Pack some of your favorite high carbohydrate snacks. Try to stay away from unusual foods to avoid any gastric surprises on race day.

Criterium Racing

Criterium or circuit races are exciting to watch—they are often shorter in length than road races and higher in intensity. They require good bike handling skills for cornering and surges in efforts to keep up with breaks and maintain a good position during the race. You may want to allow a bit more digestion time for pre-race eating, probably at least three hours. Pre-hydrate starting forty-eight hours beforehand, as drinking during criterium racing can be challenging. If the race is longer than one hour, keep a sports drink in your water bottle. Drink whenever the opportunity presents itself, and become accustomed to drinking at higher intensities. Practice recovery nutrition after criterium racing, and make sure that you consume sodium and fluid after racing in hot weather.

Time Trials

Time trials also require rest and adequate consumption of carbohydrates. Your competition efforts will require much mental concentration, focus and steady state exercise in the crouched position. A full stomach could interfere with being comfortable in this position. Allow yourself at least two to three hours of digestion time. Rest and consume adequate carbohydrates at least twenty-four hours prior to the time trial. Pre-hydrate and consume a sports drink leading up to your start time for a 40-kilometer individual time trial and 50- to 100-kilometer team time trials. You can consider consuming only water for a 20-kilometer time trial, as maintaining blood glucose may not be as challenging with the proper pre-race meal safely digested in your system. Make sure that your stomach does not get too bloated, and consume your fluid in sips. Consume fluid as efficiently as possible during the time trial. Practice consuming fluids in the crouched position. Sports drinks should be used for efforts lasting longer than one hour. You may want to try a bladder hydration system that will allow you to hold a more steady position on the bike while drinking. Rehydrate and practice recovery nutrition after your time trial.

Mountain Bike Racing

Mountain bike racing is performed on varying terrain and includes climbs, descents and challenging single-track sections. Races are often performed on a circuit, and racers will complete a specific number of laps depending on their race category. Start times are generally staggered throughout the day. Time your pre-race meal carefully, and be aware that your stomach can experience more jostling during a mountain bike race. Focus on consuming adequate carbohydrates, sodium, and fluid the day before, the night before, and the morning of the race. After your pre-race meal, about three hours beforehand, consume one to two bottles of a sports drink.

Drinking during mountain bike races is more difficult than during road races. In many sections of the race it may be impossible to let go of the handlebars. Make a conscious effort to drink during gradual climbs, dirt roads, and paved sections of the course. When you are descending or climbing over rough terrain, you will be less inclined to drink. Many mountain-bike racers use a bladder hydration system, as there is no need to let go of the handlebars when carrying one. These systems provide adequate fluid for the first one to two laps, after which you can consume a sports drink from a water bottle or have a helpful friend pass a bottle in the feed zone. Aim for consumption of one bottle per lap, or commit to certain amount of fluid per lap. Stick to the plan as closely as possible to consume 30–60 grams of carbohydrates per hour from a sports drink. For longer races you may want to consume a carbohydrate gel, but during hot races keeping up with your fluid needs is essential. If you are competing in a twenty-four-hour mountain bike race as part of a team, make sure that you practice recovery nutrition guidelines after each leg to replenish muscle glycogen. Eat a small easily digested meal if tolerated and as time allows.

Cyclo-cross

While cyclo-cross training may require some adjustments in nutrition due to very high intensity sessions and training twice daily, the most important nutritional considerations of cyclo-cross take place twenty-four hours before start time.

Though cyclo-cross race times may last only forty-five to sixty minutes, it would be prudent to optimize your muscle glycogen stores the day before a race. Because of the high-intensity level of cyclo-cross racing, a high rate of muscle glycogen depletion can result. Normalize muscle glycogen stores with twenty-four hours of rest or light training and adequate carbohydrate consumption. Avoid training sessions close to race day that will result in muscle damage, as muscle glycogen storage will be impaired. If you are competing twice over the weekend, practice good recovery nutrition after the first race.

With pre-race meal timing it is best to err on the side of caution and allow plenty of time for digestion in order to avoid "cross-gut." Pre-race nerves may further accentuate gastrointestinal upset. Most cross racers prefer to allow three to four hours of digestion time and focus on easy-to-digest carbohydrate foods. If your race begins after noon, factor in two pre-race meals. Have a large breakfast and a small "lunch" three hours prior that consists mainly of carbohydrate-based breakfast foods. Drink plenty of fluids several hours before the race for optimal hydration. Many seasoned cyclo-cross racers prefer to stop fluids thirty minutes before the race to avoid feeling bloated and miserable on the bike. Gels and sports bars can also be consumed in the two hours before race time if well tolerated.

Once you arrive at the start line, your nutritional options are likely to remain limited as cyclo-cross racing is done without a water bottle cage. Many racers try a carbohydrate gel at the start line or halfway through the race for a carbohydrate boost, as the risk of bonking during cyclo-cross seems to be high. Even with a bottle hand-up once a lap, you may be able to manage only a few gulps of fluid.

NUTRITION FOR THE RECREATIONAL CYCLIST

Many recreational cyclists ride a significant number of weekly miles, though they may exercise at lower intensities than cyclists preparing for competition. Overall, your diet should emphasize carbohydrates so that you can replenish muscle glycogen stores depleted from longer rides. After very long rides, recovery nutrition

Nutrition at High Altitude

It is possible that cyclists may live, train, or compete at altitude. Breathing at high elevations can be challenging, as can exercising. The higher the elevation, the less dense the air that you breathe. This effects results in altitude "hypoxia" or a reduction of oxygen in your body tissues. Fortunately your body adjusts or "acclimatizes" to altitude, though this process can take up to three weeks. When you travel quickly to altitude, you may experience symptoms such as rapid heart rate, headache, shortness of breath, fatigue, nausea and vomiting, loss of appetite, decreased urine output, and insomnia, often referred to as acute mountain sickness (AMS). This complex of symptoms is most likely to occur in individuals who reside at sea level and ascend rapidly to high altitude. Symptoms normally develop in six to twelve hours, peak at twenty-four to forty-eight hours, and subside in three to seven days as your body acclimatizes to altitude.

As you adjust to altitude, your blood volume will return to normal after an initial drop designed to concentrate your red blood cells that carry oxygen in your blood. You will also develop more red blood cells if you stay longer at altitude, and your muscles will begin to extract more oxygen from your blood. Altitude clearly has metabolic adaptations that affect your nutritional needs. Even relatively moderate elevations of up to 5,000 feet can affect how you should eat and drink.

The air at altitude is extremely dry, and every breath you take results in fluid loss. You also have increased "insensible" fluid losses through your skin. Normally these insensible fluid losses are about 0.5 quart daily, but can increase to 2.0 quarts daily. But your fluid needs don't stop there, as urinary losses are 1–2 quarts daily. You can also lose 2 quarts of fluid per hour during exercise.

Replacing your fluid losses must be a very conscious effort at altitude. Always try to keep some source of fluid with you. You may require 4–8 quarts of fluid daily depending on your training schedule. Avoid alcohol completely, and try to minimize caffeine intake in order to preserve fluid status. Clear urine indicates that you are matching your fluid losses.

When at altitude, you also have to consider your carbohydrate and calorie intake. Your basal metabolic rate can increase by as much as 40 percent the first few days at altitude and then drop off to about 15 percent above sea level values. Overall, your energy needs at altitude may increase by 200–300 calories daily. While this may sound like a simple calorie increase, the real decrease in appetite

that sets in at altitude may be a problem, and it may be possible to under-eat by several hundred calories daily. Undereating and losing weight at altitude does not result in body fat loss. What is more likely to occur is that your body will utilize valuable protein stores instead.

It is best if the extra calories that you eat at altitude come from carbohydrates. High carbohydrate diets may reduce the effects of acute mountain sickness. Delaying the depletion of muscle glycogen also supports endurance training improvements at altitude. Carbo hydrates are more easily digested and better tolerated than high fat foods at altitude. Keep these foods handy and have snacks to meet the additional caloric requirements. Small, frequent meals may be better tolerated with the decrease in appetite. Bonking can also creep up on you at altitude, making adequate intake of

(continued on page 234)

(continued from page 233) glucose during exercise imperative. Sports drinks clearly provide both needed fluids and carbohydrates.

While research on vitamin and mineral requirements at altitude is limited, iron is a nutrient that undoubtedly deserves your attention at higher elevations. Athletes training at altitude should have iron status monitored regularly. Having adequate iron stores ensures that you meet the demands of producing more red blood cells at altitude. Iron is an important part of hemoglobin, the component of red blood cells that carries oxygen in your body. Besides emphasizing good food sources of iron, iron supplementation may boost and maintain iron stores. Be careful not to supplement to excess, and do so under a physician's supervision. Too much iron causes oxidation and free radical production.

Focusing on foods high in antioxidants like vitamins C and E may also be beneficial, as exercising at high altitude places "oxidative stress" upon your body. Exercise at altitude may also raise your vitamin E requirements. Food sources include fortified cereals, whole grains, wheat germ, nuts and seeds, green leafy vegetables, and vegetable oils. Recommendations for vitamin E supplementation are currently at 100–400 IU daily. ■

is helpful for replenishing and minimizing your fatigue over the next several days. If you ride after work or commute, make sure that you always carry adequate fluid and focus on hydration both on and off the bike. Clear urine indicates that you are well hydrated.

When preparing for longer weekend rides including centuries, you may want to rest twenty-four to forty-eight hours prior and focus on consuming a diet higher in carbohydrates in order to fill up your muscle glycogen stores. Focus on eating a meal high in carbohydrates several hours before the ride to fill up liver glycogen stores. When you ride longer than ninety minutes, even at lower intensities, make an effort to consume 30–60 grams of carbohydrates per hour from sports drinks to maintain hydration and blood glucose levels. Because you may be riding at relatively lower intensities, consuming solid foods and gels during the ride along with water may be relatively simple and enjoyable. Organized rides also have fuel stops where you will find water, fresh fruit, and other easily digested carbohydrates. You can also pack some of your favorite on-bike foods and store them in your jersey pockets and in various bike bag options. Experimentation will teach you what foods work best for your stomach. It is best to start refueling early to prevent hypoglycemia. If you do start to manifest some of the symptoms of hypoglycemia, slow down and take in some carbohydrates.

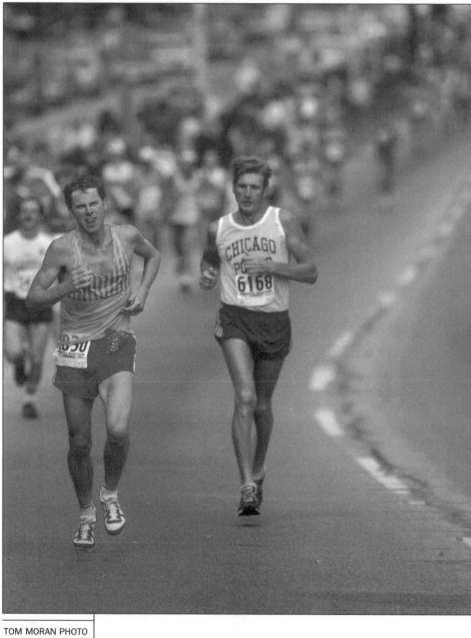

TOM MORAN PHOTO

chapter 11

NUTRITION FOR DISTANCE RUNNING

The number of athletes participating in the sport of running currently stands at an all-time high. Running has also broadened in scope. It is not only for the lean and elite, but now includes masters runners of a wide range of ages, slower runners, heavier runners, and everyday runners training for their first marathon. It is estimated that the number of marathon entrants in the U.S. now exceeds 400,000 yearly. In fact the average running time for the marathon is getting longer, reflecting how the scope of participation in this race has expanded. The largest age groups at the races are now men in their late thirties and early forties and women in their twenties. Runners are highly likely to be club members, train with a coach, and enter events that raise money for charity.

Distance runners compete over a variety of race lengths. Some of the most common distances include 10K (6.2 miles), 15K (9.3 miles), half-marathons (21.1K or 13.1 miles), and the marathon (42.2K or 26.2 miles). There are also ultradistance events, such as 50K (31 miles), 100K (62 miles), and 100-mile events, which do not attract as large a number of participants, especially at the recreational level. Distance runners tend to improve their performance with age, and many run and train for more than a decade before they reach their best running times. Many runners are often simply satisfied to run for optimal fitness and health and also enjoy the social aspects of running.

TRAINING NUTRITION

Running is a broad sport in that runners may compete in a variety of distances during the year, and from one to dozens of races. Even an experienced marathoner may choose to compete in an early season 10K race, half-marathon, and perhaps one marathon a season. Recreational runners may train for their first marathon and join a fundraising organization. Because of the broad range of competitive goals, training programs are somewhat specific to the athlete. Running sessions include longer runs designed to develop aerobic endurance and intense runs and interval work designed to improve the anaerobic system and speed.

Daily training sessions for a 10K may consist of thirty to sixty minutes of running, a long run, and fast runs. Upping the competitive distance to a half-marathon as your race goal will increase the length of your base training runs and the distance of your long run. You may incorporate a 5K or 10K race into your training plan. Marathon training requires months of preparation, with carefully scheduled long runs and time for adequate recovery. Weekly marathon training can approach 30–45 miles weekly. Elite marathon runners may train twice daily and up to 90 miles weekly. Water running or weight training may also be included in a runner's program.

Pre-exercise Eating

Eating too much and eating too close to training or competition are probably the biggest nutritional mistakes that a runner can make. Because running jostles your stomach and gastrointestinal system, GI disturbance is a more common problem than in other endurance sports. Timing your pre-exercise meals is important for feeling "light" during your run and avoiding unpleasant symptoms such as a sloshing stomach and bloating.

Prior to shorter easy runs, what you eat before training may simply be a matter of comfort and fending off hunger or hypoglycemia. It is not uncommon for runners to train in the early morning hours, and they often forgo a pre-exercise snack when training later in the day. Some runners experiment and choose to have something light such as juice and a plain piece of toast before an early morning run. Regardless of your tolerances, make sure that you drink water to hydrate. If you have some early morning long runs planned, consider taking a water bottle with you. During steady state endurance running, you may want to consume a sports drink. It is good practice for longer races and maintains blood glucose levels in the latter part of the run.

Consuming regular meals and snacks does replenish your more labile liver glycogen stores and consequently helps maintain steady blood glucose levels throughout the day and during training. For afternoon or evening runs, try to time your meals carefully and eat three or more hours before running. Leave enough space between meal or snack times and training times before higher intensity runs and speedwork. Emphasize carbohydrate sources that are easily digested. You may want to consider a liquid sports supplement or meal replacement before longer training sessions.

Experiment with pre-race eating before your weekend long run. This practice sets the stage for knowing your tolerances and preferences on race day. While it may be tempting to sleep in before long runs, the pre-exercise meal is important for filling both liver and muscle glycogen stores. Liquid meals may work best, but you can also experiment with carbohydrate foods low in fiber. Knowing what works for you in training will help lighten pre-race nerves and make you more comfortable about your nutritional choices on the big day.

Hydration and Fluids

Runners should focus on consuming fluids throughout the day and maintaining adequate hydration. Clear urine indicates that you are well hydrated. Try to consume at least 8–12 ounces every hour when not training. Practice the pre-hydration guidelines outlined in Chapter 5. Find the best timing to prevent sloshing in your stomach during training.

Recovery Nutrition

Training, particularly hard and twice-daily sessions, require that you pay attention to recovery nutrition. Running can also cause some damage to muscle fibers, which can delay glycogen recovery. Carbohydrate intake immediately after training will start the process of muscle glycogen resynthesis and prevent the gradual process of muscle glycogen depletion that can occur over several days or longer. Consume 50–100 grams of carbohydrates immediately after exercise and plenty of fluids for recovery. Monitor weight before and after running and consume 24 ounces of fluid for every pound lost. You can also emphasize sources of sodium after training sessions to improve the rehydration process, particularly after training in hot weather. Make sure that you continue to rehydrate the rest of the day, and use weight as a gauge of hydration. Remember that thirst is not the most sensitive indicator of fluid needs. Carry fluid with you everywhere you go and drink constantly.

Weight Management

Elite distance runners are typically lean, most likely due to having a body type appropriate for their sport and their high volume of training. However, many runners are aware that carrying "dead weight" does not enhance performance. What is essential for serious runners to appreciate is that they should aim for a target weight that is not unrealistically low and that can be maintained without excessive training or stringent dieting. An overtrained or underfed runner does not produce his best performance. It is best to focus on sensible weight loss strategies such as those outlined in Chapter 7.

The Importance of Iron

Distance runners, especially females, seem to be at higher risk for developing compromised iron status. If untreated, iron deficiency can lead to anemia, which clearly impairs exercise performance. But even iron deficiency appears to affect training and performance in some athletes. Clearly, iron deficiency needs to be corrected before it progresses into anemia.

Iron deficiency should be treated with a diet high in heme iron. Good sources are listed in Table 3.7, but include lean red meat, chicken, and fish. Non-heme iron can also be emphasized and consumed with a food source of vitamin C to enhance absorption. You can consume iron-fortified cereal with orange juice, mix beans and tomatoes in dishes such as chili, and include a baked potato and broccoli at the same meal. Iron fortified breads and cereals are also a major source of iron in the diet. If you purchase natural foods that are not iron fortified, you may reduce your iron intake by emphasizing these food sources. To maximize your iron absorption from foods, do not consume them with foods that inhibit iron absorption such as coffee, tea, and excessive intakes of bran. Bran products contain phytates, which inhibit iron absorption. Phytates are also found in nuts, seeds, wheat cereals, peanut butter, and soy products. If you don't eat adequate amounts of heme iron, consider taking a low dose iron supplement as part of a multivitamin providing 15 milligrams of iron daily.

It makes sense for runners, especially females, to screen for iron deficiency once yearly. Low levels of serum ferritin may warrant safe and monitored supplementation to bring levels back up into the middle range. Occasionally, increases in serum ferritin result in a slight increase in hemoglobin, reflecting that a mild anemia may have been present. It is also possible that an athlete can benefit from a slightly higher level of hemoglobin, and may have his or her own individual "normal" range for optimal performance.

An iron treatment dose is often more than 50 milligrams daily, and up to 300 milligrams daily for more severe anemia, but don't start taking therapeutic iron doses without first seeing a physician. Some individuals are susceptible to hemochromatosis, or iron overload, in which excess iron is deposited in the liver and other internal organs, causing serious damage. Too much iron when it is not really required can also decrease absorption of other important minerals like copper and zinc. Also, don't self-diagnose an iron deficiency when feeling run-down and tired. Fatigue can be related to a number of health, nutritional, and training factors.

Body Weight, Amenorrhea, and Bone Density

Bone health is an issue that has received heightened attention over the past two decades due to the increasing rate of osteoporotic fractures and a focus on stress fractures. The athlete at risk for development of compromised bone health should appreciate the influence of exercise, hormone balance, and nutritional factors such as calcium intake on maintaining appropriate levels of this important body tissue.

Bone is a dynamic tissue that is constantly being broken down and rebuilt under the regulation of your body's hormones. When the process of bone breakdown or bone resorption exceeds bone formation, bone loss occurs. If this bone loss is prolonged, osteoporosis, a condition in which low bone mass has developed and bone is fragile, can result, and there is greater risk for fracture. Calcium balance is maintained by the amount of calcium you consume and absorb, and how much calcium you lose in your urine. The hormone estrogen plays a crucial role in maintaining bone in women. When estrogen levels are low, the bone serves as a source of calcium to maintain normal levels of calcium in the blood and perform important physiological functions in the body. Even if physical activity is high, low estrogen levels as seen in amenorrhea and after menopause can result in bone loss. Female athletes seem to have a higher incidence of menstrual irregularities than the general female population. Genetics also has a large influence on your bone density.

The term "athletic amenorrhea" has been used to describe menstrual imbalances in female athletes. A variety of factors have been implicated in the development of amenorrhea in athletes. It appears that the predominant factor in development of amenorrhea is inadequate energy intake. An excessive training load or increase in training that is not matched with proper food intake creates a caloric deficiency that can result in amenorrhea. Of course, disordered eating and a full-blown eating disorder can also result in chronically low intake of calories. Amenorrhea may also be more common in certain sports such as running, gymnastics, and dance.

What has been determined is that female athletes with amenorrhea have lower bone mass than athletes who menstruate regularly. Greater incidence of stress fractures has also been reported in athletes with current or past menstrual disturbances. Athletes with these health concerns should see a sports medicine physician for assessment of bone mass and hormonal status and seek appropriate medical treatment.

Athletes being treated for amenorrhea should increase their calcium intake to 1,500 milligrams daily. Refer to Chapter 3 for a list of foods high in calcium. If this amount cannot be achieved through diet, calcium supplements can make up the difference. Doses of 500 milligrams of calcium carbonate or calcium citrate can be taken one to two times daily. Excessive protein, when combined with inadequate calcium intake and high intakes of caffeine and sodium, can also aggravate calcium absorption. Overall balance in the diet, especially adequate calorie intake, should also be restored. Weight-bearing exercise may also be continued, though not at excessive levels. ■

When you have true anemia, a physician can prescribe a therapeutic dose of iron. Liquid ferrous sulfate is well absorbed. You can increase your dose slowly to minimize any gastrointestinal side effects of taking the supplement. Ferrous gluconate is often better tolerated than other forms of iron. Take your supplement on an empty stomach with a dose of vitamin C or a glass of orange juice. Iron supplements should be taken separately from calcium supplements to prevent a decrease in iron absorption. Your physician can monitor your serum ferritin and hemoglobin levels for several months afterward and continue, adjust, or discontinue supplementation as appropriate.

COMPETITION NUTRITION

Competition in running is primarily an aerobic activity with elite runners completing a 10K in less than thirty minutes and recreational runners taking twice as long to complete the same distance. Elite marathoners race just over two hours, while recreational runners may take more than five hours to complete a marathon. Many marathons also include walkers who enter for fundraising purposes and take even longer to complete the 26.2-mile event. Hydration is critical for all events, and races lasting longer than ninety minutes clearly challenge your body's carbohydrate stores.

10K Race

Because of the relatively short time in which it will be completed, a 10K race is unlikely to challenge your muscle glycogen stores, though your liver glycogen stores may be a bit low in the morning. A pre-race meal can help keep blood glucose levels nice and steady through your warm-up and race, and prevent feelings of hunger. Of course you will want to be cautious when choosing your pre-race foods and your meal timing. Experiment in training with timing and portions, and consume easily digested carbohydrate foods and/or liquids that you know you can tolerate.

Your major nutritional risk during a race of this length will be dehydration. Faster runners competing in cool weather are unlikely to waste time to stop and drink. But as race times and the temperature increase, adequate fluid intake remains essential prior to racing to prevent dehydration from developing. You require fluid when you wake up in the morning and can lose fluid in the hours prior to the race through sweating and urination. You may want to try experimenting with a sports drink for both fluid and a carbohydrate boost before racing a 10K and sip it in the time before the race. Carbohydrate sensitive athletes can experiment with this pre-race strategy in training. Just make sure that you allow yourself plenty of time to empty your bladder before racing. Fluid intake during the race may benefit racers running for more than an hour. Stick with about 2–3 cups of fluid total spread out over the race. You may want to consume only water, but a sports drink may also be appealing and well tolerated.

Half-marathon and Marathon

For some competitors, the half-marathon does not present significant challenges to tapping into stored fuel as top runners complete the race in less than ninety minutes. However, the vast majority of runners will complete the half-marathon in more than ninety minutes, and perhaps in two to three hours. What matters is that you are aware of your projected race time and plan your nutrition program leading up to the race accordingly. If the race will significantly impact your carbohydrate stores, you need to maximize these fuel reserves prior to the race. Plan your pre-race meal and emphasize easily digested carbohydrate foods. Liquid sources low in fiber should be well tolerated. Aim to consume 30–60 grams of carbohydrates during the race for times lasting longer than ninety minutes. Sports drinks are generally the best-tolerated source of carbohydrates. Many runners have also experimented successfully with gels as their source of carbohydrates.

Clearly the marathon presents nutritional challenges to even the most elite competitors. Lasting more than two hours for the world's top runners, hitting the wall or running low on muscle glycogen at the 20-mile mark is a real possibility, as this race uses up all the muscle glycogen you can store and then some.

Carbohydrate loading is synonymous with the marathon. The principals of carbohydrate loading and the most current research-based guidelines are provided in

Chapter 5. After your last long run prior to the marathon, pay extra close attention to matching or even slightly exceeding your carbohydrate requirements for the remainder of your training during taper week. For maximum glycogen stores, an intake of 4–5 grams carbohydrates per pound of weight has been recommended, or about 500–700 grams daily. However, carbohydrate loading does not necessarily require enormous amounts of food and calories. On rest days your calorie needs may not be especially high, and you simply need to eat enough carbohydrate to fill up your glycogen stores. This may only require that a greater percentage of your calories is derived from carbohydrates, preferably those low in fiber.

During this critical time, make sure that non-carbohydrate foods do not crowd out foods high in carbohydrates. Exceeding your protein and fat requirements serves little purpose the forty-eight hours before the marathon. Just make certain to keep reasonable amounts of protein and fat in your diet. Have a menu prepared ahead of time to ensure that you not only choose high carbohydrate foods, but also that you consume enough of them. Refer to the food lists providing 30-gram carbohydrate servings, and draw out some sample meals. Beware of sweet foods that may provide some carbohydrate but also plenty of fat. They may fill you up and taste good, but they won't fill up your muscle glycogen stores adequately. This may also be a good time period in which to consume some extra sugar and high carbohydrate fluids such as juices and smoothies that also have the added bonus of being low in fiber. You may wish to avoid very high fiber foods twenty-four to forty-eight hours before the event to "race light" and reduce gastrointestinal contents. Some runners have even dropped one or two pounds by reducing fiber in the diet several days before the race.

It is important that you are aware that your body stores a considerable amount of fluid when you carbohydrate load. Don't be alarmed if your muscles feel a bit stiff or the number on your weight scale increases when carbohydrate loading. This additional stored water helps to delay dehydration during the race. Of course you should also hydrate your body by drinking plenty of fluids in the forty-eight hours prior to the race. Keep a water bottle and hydrating fluids with you at all times. Monitor the color of your urine to ensure that it is clear and that you are adequately hydrated.

Plan to consume a high carbohydrate breakfast the morning of the race. You can somewhat diminish overnight liver glycogen losses by consuming a late evening snack. However, this pre-race meal is much more effective at refilling liver glycogen and helping you maintain blood glucose levels when racing, when compared to not eating the morning of the race. Eating breakfast also settles your stomach and prevents hunger while racing. Some runners may prefer to have a liquid meal replacement or breakfast shake in order to avoid solid food before several hours of hard running. Experiment during longer runs to determine your favorite and best-tolerated pre-race meal. If you are traveling to the race, you may want to pack some of your favorite race foods to supplement your restaurant diet. Avoid trying new foods in the days leading up to the race. If you will be running in hotter weather, or for several hours, increase your salt intake prior to the race to prevent a decrease in blood sodium levels while racing.

What you consume during the marathon is just as important as what you had beforehand. Fluid needs are also crucial. The faster you run, the more heat you produce and the greater your risk of dehydration. While many marathons start in the early morning to avoid excess heat, it is possible that you will complete your run in hotter temperatures. Running longer than ninety minutes will also challenge your body's carbohydrate stores no matter how careful your pre-race eating.

Focus early in the race on consuming carbohydrates in order to delay depletion of your glycogen stores. Sports drinks are your best-tolerated option and provide both needed fluid and carbohydrates. Energy gels are another option favored by marathoners. Make sure to wash them down with 6–8 ounces of water.

Aid stations are generally provided every mile. Find out ahead of time what sports drink will be provided at the race and drink it during training to develop a taste and tolerance to the product. You need to average about 4 to 8 ounces every fifteen to twenty minutes. Practice drinking and running in shorter early season races. Even seasoned racers do not consume the full amount of liquid provided in the cup, but you can practice your technique. Pinch the cup to form a funnel and take down two gulps. If you have to slow up in order to drink, you will still improve your race time by consuming adequate fluid and carbohydrates.

Many runners also consume carbohydrate gels during a marathon. Make sure that you consume a gel packet with 8 ounces of water. If you think that you will require several energy gels during the race, consider carrying them in a waistband or waist pack. Your goal is to consume at least 30–60 grams of carbohydrates every hour.

Runner's Diarrhea

Runners seem to be more susceptible than other endurance athletes to gastrointestinal distress and diarrhea during training and racing, as the constant jarring and repetitive motion of running may aggravate your colon. GI upset may also be related to the intensity of your running, decreased blood flow to the GI tract, and dehydration. Some runners may also be able to identify specific foods that aggravate GI problems.

Drink plenty of fluids before and during exercise to prevent dehydration and maintain adequate blood flow to your intestinal system. Start drinking early to prevent dehydration. Some runners have benefited from lowering their fiber intake close to exercise. You may even want to reduce your fiber intake at dinner, prior to early morning runs the next day. Caffeine, particularly from coffee, is known to have a laxative effect. Avoid it, as well as the artificial sweeteners sorbitol and aspartame, which may also aggravate symptoms. Make sure that you are not taking any medications or over-the-counter supplements that aggravate GI symptoms, and eliminate the possibility of intestinal parasites. ■

Practice these nutrition strategies during training. Don't make plain water your major source of fluid during the race. Slower runners are especially at risk for developing hyponatremia. Consuming mainly plain water over several hours does not adequately replace sodium losses during exercise. Therefore, runners who will take several hours to complete the race are at greater risk for developing low sodium blood levels.

By race day, you should have mastered the best fluid and fuel replacement techniques that support your individual preferences and tolerances. You should also be flexible enough to consume the products offered on race day and adjust your plan as needed during the race.

Ultrarunning

Ultradistance races typically start at distances of 31 miles, but can also be 50, 62, and 100 miles. Other races are organized around a time frame where you run as far as possible for twelve, twenty-four, and forty-eight hours. Clearly for races of such length, nutrition is an important factor in completing the race. Runners training for ultras extend the weekly long run that is the core of marathon training. Besides building stamina and mental fortitude, the longer runs also give you the opportunity to develop eating and drinking skills.

For competition, the taper presents the opportunity to carbohydrate load as discussed under the marathon plan. Eat a large snack the night before the race, and have your tried and true pre-race breakfast already planned out and tested. Use liquid supplements as needed and hyperhydrate before the race. Increase your salt intake to compensate for salt losses during the race.

Dehydration is the main culprit that prevents a runner from completing an ultra race. Drink at least 20 ounces of fluid per hour. Set your watch if you need to remind yourself to drink. Carry a sports drink for both carbohydrates and fluids. Have a predetermined fluid schedule outlined, and keep a specific number of bottles available at each aid station. Experiment with other supplements such as gels, energy bars, and liquid meals to determine what you tolerate while running.

You may find fruit, pretzels, cookies, and baked potatoes at aid stations. Practice with these foods during training. Take along some tolerated salty food items and salt tablets to replace sodium losses during the race.

Start replacing fluid, carbohydrates, and sodium early, so that you can finish the race. Once you become depleted, it can be difficult to dig yourself out of a nutritional hole. If your stomach feels bloated and is not emptying properly, you may be dehydrated. If your stomach does become overfull and you vomit, start consuming a sports drink slowly afterward to rehydrate. It will empty from your stomach as quickly as water and provide needed carbohydrates and sodium.

Sodium losses vary greatly among individuals and in various weather conditions. Experiment in training with use of salt tablets to determine what works for you. Salty foods such as soup or broth may also be available at aid stations for some electrolyte replenishment. Keep any salt tablets that you carry with you away from moisture so that they do not break down before you ingest them. Wrapping them in plastic should work. Make sure that you ingest salt tablets with plenty of water. If you determine that you are losing weight during the race at check-ins, rehydrate with sodium-containing fluids that increase fluid retention.

Drinking your calories is still your best option. Experiment with various drinks and flavors to prevent taste fatigue. Try to consume more than 250 calories per hour. Besides sports drinks, you may benefit from more concentrated sources such as high carbohydrate supplements and meal replacements. These products will not be as hydrating but provide needed carbohydrates. Make sure that you consume them when you are keeping up with your hydration needs. Have a variety of foods available along the way. It is fine if you decide not to have them, but they can provide some variety and satisfy a craving along the way. Caffeinated soft drinks can provide an energy and mental boost later in the race. Time your eating and drinking when you slow down to a walk, usually when you are going uphill.

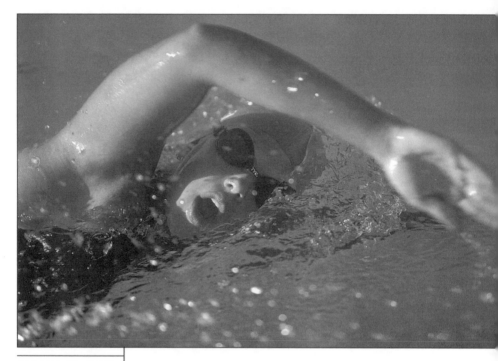

DAN CAMPBELL PHOTO

chapter 12

NUTRITION FOR SWIMMING

I ndividuals of all ages and abilities are involved in the sport of swimming. Swimmers train with local clubs, on high school teams, and in college. Age-group swimming starts at age ten and continues through high school. The National Collegiate Athletic Association (NCAA) has a strong swimming program. United States Masters Swimming offers training and competition opportunities for athletes ranging from 19 to 100 years old and includes more than 40,000 members in the U.S. Many masters teams train at local YMCA pools or high school and university pools. Competitive swimming also includes open water swimming.

NUTRITION FOR TRAINING

Swim training programs can vary greatly depending on the swimmer's age, fitness level, competitive goals, and race events and distances. Master swimmers may train at high intensities and anywhere from one to two hours daily. Collegiate swim training is often very demanding and in sharp contrast to the brevity of the competitive events for which these swimmers train. Though swimming requires highly specific training, collegiate swimmers often include weight training and land training such as running or cycling in their programs. Masters swimmers also frequently participate in weight training, cycling, and running, and many members compete in triathlons. The number of hours of weekly training varies greatly among masters swimmers, but often comprises enough weekly training hours to warrant paying proper attention to an endurance training diet.

For serious swimmers, training may include two sessions daily, in the early morning and afternoon or evening to accommodate school and work schedules. The total number of weekly sessions can vary with training level, competitive goals, and the stage of the season. Very serious swimmers may complete twelve sessions per week for a total of two to four hours daily, and up to twenty hours weekly. Non-collegiate swimmers may train both in and out of water for a total of eight to twelve hours weekly. Swim training workout intensities can vary greatly and include both aerobic and endurance base training. Swimming also includes a number of anaerobic training sessions of interval work at different percentages of maximal heart rates.

Clearly, swim training programs consist of workouts that can rely heavily on muscle glycogen stores for fuel. Swimmers who do not replenish these stores after harder training sessions may find that they eventually are unable to complete subsequent sessions due to inadequate recovery. Even swimmers who frequently crosstrain for a variety of athletic goals and basic convenience may find that their total training hours accumulate and necessitate the benefits afforded by proper endurance nutrition. Technique is also an important consideration in becoming a successful swimmer.

It is interesting to note that swimming competition generally lasts from dozens of seconds to dozens of minutes, making competition highly anaerobic, though aerobic metabolism becomes more significant as the distance of the event increases. Because of these relatively short race times at high intensities, swimming competition requires its own set of nutritional strategies as build-up of lactic acid, rather than depletion of fuel stores, is likely to be the limiting performance factor. Of course an exception would be long distance swimming, which requires athletes to compete in much longer events and which has a smaller following than other swim categories. Regardless of the competitive event, training, and particularly serious training, requires that you pay close attention to nutrition guidelines prescribed to endurance athletes.

Recovery Nutrition

Calories and Carbohydrates

Calorie requirements for swimming increase as the volume and intensity of the individual training sessions and total program increase. Because of the wide range of training programs found among swimmers of all ages and competitive levels, refer to the calorie levels outlined in Chapter 4. Your calorie requirements can vary day to day, depending on the intensity and distance of your swim and crosstraining efforts. Review these recommendations to determine what training days necessitate higher intakes for optimal recovery. Pay close attention to eating well during successive heavier training days so that fatigue and a subpar performance do not halt training at week's end. Younger swimmers require adequate calories for both growth and training, and are likely to consume many calories, though daily caloric needs of Olympic swimmers can exceed several thousand. Swimming may burn anywhere from 500 to 700 calories per hour.

Of course adequate calorie intake is synonymous with consuming enough total grams of carbohydrates for optimal recovery. Swim training typically lasts from 60 to 120 minutes per session. Shorter sessions of high intensity interval or speedwork training can also deplete muscle glycogen stores. Longer steady state sessions, by the nature of their duration, also utilize this important and limited fuel supply. Match up your daily carbohydrate intake with your training as outlined in Table 4.3. After strenuous training sessions, consume adequate carbohydrates for recovery. Aim for 0.5 grams of carbohydrates per pound of weight, or about 50–75 grams of carbohydrates immediately after exercise to begin the synthesis of muscle glycogen before the next training session. You can also combine this carbohydrate with small amounts of protein if desired, but make sure carbohydrate intake is your first priority. Convenient items that can be brought to the pool for consumption include energy bars, high carbohydrate supplements, bagels, crackers, juices, and fruit.

Fluid Requirements

Swimmers are in the unique position of both sweating in water and exercising in cool temperatures, rendering sweat loss from the swim an elusive and difficult measurement. The question that sports scientists would like to definitively answer is just how much athletes sweat in water. Because being in water can actually cool the body, swimmers may not need to sweat as much to dissipate heat produced during training. Warm pool water, warm air temperature, and humidity can still affect the hydration levels of swimmers, particularly in an outdoor pool.

Limited data currently indicate that sweat losses in the pool are relatively moderate when compared to other types of endurance training, even when you spend a significant amount of time traveling up and down the pool. Though these sweat losses are not as heavy as those measured in cyclists or triathletes, they should be replaced with fluid intake during training. As in any sport, one of the best techniques for monitoring your fluid losses is to weigh yourself before and after training. Every pound of weight lost represents the need to drink 24 ounces of fluid to replace sweat and subsequent urine losses. Keep in mind that sweat rates vary among individual athletes. Though the average fluid losses among swimmers may be relatively moderate when compared to land athletes who train in the heat, some individuals may have higher sweat rates.

Fortunately, swim training presents a convenient opportunity to replace sweat losses, whether modest or significant. Leave your water bottle at the end or your lane for longer or more intense swim sessions. Concentrate on taking gulps every fifteen minutes or so or when the nature of the training session allows you to drink without disrupting interval work. Gauge if your drinking habits are keeping up with your losses by weighing yourself before and after training. Assess how well you achieve fluid balance for various types of training sessions. You may even want to check that you don't overhydrate. Because sweat losses are somewhat diminished when swimming, very motivated drinkers may even exceed their fluid losses. For training sessions exceeding one hour, and for shorter sessions that are high in intensity, consume a sports drink. These drinks provide carbohydrates to maintain adequate blood glucose levels and supply your muscles with fuel when body stores run low. Sports drinks can easily meet both your carbohydrate and fluid requirements if consumed in adequate amounts. They also increase the drive to drink and enhance fluid absorption. Aim for 20–30 ounces of a sports drink every hour. Drink immediately before and after practice and between swim sets.

MASTERS SWIMMING

Masters swimming encompasses athletes ranging in age from 19 to 100 years. Men and women are eligible to swim masters regardless of ability, speed, age, or competitive swimming background. A wide variety of events are offered at swim meets including freestyle events ranging from 50 to 1,500 meters, and 50-, 100-, and 200-meter distances for freestyle, backstroke, breaststroke, and butterfly. Relay events are also offered, as are open water distance events longer than 1 mile and up to 10 kilometers.

When surveyed by USMS, masters swimmers indicated that they swim anywhere from two to six days weekly. Most USMS members weight train regularly and cycle and run to complement their swimming. Probably one of the most significant physiological changes that occur with aging is a slight decrease in muscle mass after age 30. Resistance or weight training can offset these muscle losses and provide the masters athlete with the benefits of maintaining strength and power, and building muscle, which is metabolically active tissue. Weight training can also strengthen weak body areas and improve your strength-to-weight ratio. Masters athletes who are dedicated to resistance training should refer to the corresponding nutrition guidelines provided in Chapter 7.

Because of the large range of training commitments and schedules found among masters athletes, calorie and carbohydrate requirements also vary with the intensity and volume of training. Masters athletes should be aware that these nutritional requirements could change throughout the year, for seasonal adjustments in training volume and focus. As athletes age, a decrease in calories may be necessary to maintain a healthy weight. However, the quality of the diet should not be compromised, and nutrient dense foods become an even more important component of the diet when calorie requirements decrease.

Aging and the Masters Athlete

Although aging is regarded as a function of chronological age, it may be a very poor predictor of functional age. Masters athletes in their fifties and sixties can often outperform sedentary persons in their twenties. But even well conditioned and trained athletes will experience a decline in aerobic power after age 30 to 35. VO_2 max declines after age 25, but at a slower rate than in sedentary individuals. Muscle strength plateaus at ages 35–40 and then declines, though muscle strength can be maintained and improved with a good resistance training program. Masters athletes adopt healthy lifestyles and appear to derive very tangible health benefits from these good habits and their training. Benefits may include more favorable blood lipid profiles and lower risk for developing hypertension, diabetes, and osteoporosis.

Carbohydrate, protein, and fat recommendations are thought to be similar to those for younger athletes with comparable training programs. Aging may increase the need for calcium in women to prevent osteoporosis, though men can also develop this debilitating condition. Vitamin D requirements increase after age 50, as do vitamin B_6 requirements. Continuing to choose nutrient dense foods throughout a lifetime is useful for meeting increased vitamin and mineral needs with aging. Masters athletes concerned about adequate vitamin and mineral intake can take a balanced low-dose multivitamin and mineral supplement. This supplement should also provide the daily value of vitamin B_{12} for individuals over age 60. Gastric acid levels decrease with aging and don't allow B_{12} to be absorbed by the body. Calcium supplementation may also be beneficial to meet higher calcium needs.

In fact, one recent study that included men and women over age 65, conducted by researchers at Tufts University, found that an average intake of 1,350 milligrams of calcium (500 of which came from a supplement) combined with a higher protein diet produced higher bone mineral densities after three years. Lower calcium intakes of 850 milligrams daily did not work synergistically with the protein to improve bone density. Researchers are still trying to determine the underlying mechanisms and why the high protein intake did not increase calcium excretion in the urine. The bottom line from this study is not for older individuals to eat more protein but to meet their calcium requirements.

Older athletes should also pay attention to fluid intake. Thirst sensation declines in older individuals, affecting body water regulation. Fluid requirements also increase, as more water is needed to remove waste products. Generally, older athletes can tolerate exercise in the heat but should drink as much fluid as possible before and after exercise. They should aim for the high end of recommended fluid intake during exercise, consuming 8 ounces every fifteen minutes. Older athletes should pay close attention to warning signs of dehydration and be aware of how any medications may affect heat regulation. ■

HIGH SCHOOL SWIMMING

Many dedicated swimmers are in adolescence and experience dramatic physical changes in their bodies during this time. In order to reach their full growth potential, the energy demands of both growing and training must be met. This is especially true of adolescent boys who often require frequent meals and snacks in order to maintain weight and growth. They should also include high quality protein in their diet and may require up to 1.6 to 2.0 grams of protein per pound of weight. These elevated protein requirements are easily provided in a well-balanced diet, particularly if energy needs are met. Protein supplements are not necessary for a high school swimmer's diet.

Swimmers who struggle to meet caloric requirements may simply find that busy training and school schedules limit their time to eat. Planning is essential for these calorie-burning athletes. Close attention should be paid to recovery nutrition after early morning training. Packing foods and fluids high in carbohydrates is essential, as the athlete may travel to school. If the schedule and classroom setting allows, a mid-morning snack will continue the recovery process. Lunch should not be left to some fatty choice in the school cafeteria, but be planned out and consist of high quality protein, adequate carbohydrates, and reasonable amounts of good fats. A pre-exercise snack is also useful for maintaining energy levels and steady blood glucose levels for afternoon training. Of course a variety of foods is essential for a balanced diet, and young athletes should appreciate that good food choices support muscle growth, recovery, and top performance.

Adolescent swimmers should consume water during breaks in training, or sports drinks for training lasting longer than sixty minutes. Sports drinks maintain hydration levels and provide fuel for athletes who have not eaten in several hours. High intensity training sessions can also warrant the ingestion of sports drinks to provide glucose for fuel.

While consuming a high level of calories often ensures a diet adequate in vitamins and minerals, adolescents often fall short of their calcium and iron requirements. Good intakes of calcium along with training help the athlete achieve peak bone mass, reduce risk of stress fractures, and minimize the effects of bone loss later in life. Good sources of calcium as listed in Chapter 3 should be emphasized in the diet.

Iron intake may also fall short, particularly for adolescent girls who have increased iron losses with menstruation. High iron food sources are provided in

Chapter 3 and should be emphasized in the diet. A multivitamin providing the RDA for iron may be beneficial, but higher doses should not be taken without a physician's supervision.

Overall, reliance on fast-food should be minimized as much as possible to limit intake of fatty foods and hydrogenated and saturated fats. Packing fruits to supplement school lunches is an option. Low fat milk and yogurt may also be available at most school cafeterias. Athletes can pack healthy low fat lunches consisting of sandwiches, fruit, and other carbohydrate items such as pretzels and granola bars. Parents should become involved in meal planning and assist the athlete. Dinners should emphasize quality protein sources and whole grains. An evening snack can provide additional nutritious calories.

Because female adolescents experience hormonal changes leading to an increase in body fat, younger swimmers may struggle with weight management issues despite their high energy output during training. Rather than trying to conform to an ideal, female swimmers should realize that their body fat levels are likely within a healthy range. They should appreciate that success in competition is related to a number of factors and not solely on low body fat levels. Sensible strategies for controlling weight at a healthy level should be provided. Weight loss guidelines are provided in Chapter 7. It is important that extreme diets such as limiting all fat in the diet or following a very low calorie level are avoided. In some cases, rigid dieting can lead to disordered eating and full-blown eating disorders.

COLLEGIATE SWIMMING

Swimmers in college are limited by the NCAA to twenty hours of training during the regular season. Training often consists of two practice sessions daily. These athletes frequently weight train, and running is often part of their training program.

Collegiate swimmers must meet high energy and carbohydrate requirements and practice the principles of recovery nutrition, particularly when training twice daily. Inadequate carbohydrates between an early morning and late afternoon training session can compromise performance. Carbohydrates should be consumed immediately after training and should be followed by a high carbohydrate meal or snack. Carbohydrates can also be consumed several hours prior to exercise to replenish liver glycogen stores and provide fuel for the second training session. Fluid losses during training should be monitored by checking body weight before and after exercise. Water and sports drinks can be consumed during high intensity, longer duration, or strength training sessions to replace fluid and carbohydrate losses. The real challenge for collegiate athletes is meeting their nutritional requirements when eating at the college dorm or preparing meals in their own apartments.

Men and Osteoporosis

Currently, two million American men have osteoporosis and another three million are at risk for developing the disease. According to the National Osteoporosis Foundation, one-third of all hip fractures occur in men. Men also suffer from osteoporotic fractures of the spine, wrist, and other bones. Despite the fact that this disease significantly affects men, it remains underdiagnosed, underreported and inadequately treated for this gender.

It has long been known that proper exercise for stimulating osteoblasts, the cells that build bone, is weight-bearing activity and weight training. But some sports such as swimming and cycling do not offer these specific weight-bearing benefits. Swimmers and cyclists should crosstrain and weight train. Nutrition also plays a role in preventing osteoporosis in men. Men's diets seem to become calcium deficient around age 25, with two-thirds of men not meeting the recommended requirement of 1,000 milligrams (1,200 milligrams over age 50). Men should also ensure that they

Dorm Life

Eating dorm food can present challenges to the college athlete accustomed to family-style home cooked meals or having control of their own meal preparation. While athletes can keep foods in their dorm room and purchase foods on campus, the majority of their nutritional needs will be met by consuming breakfast, lunch, and dinner at the dorm food hall.

Several challenges are presented with this eating style. Eating hours are limited and must be coordinated around class and training times. These hours may not always be sufficient to accommodate heavy schedules, and the serious swimmer

consume adequate vitamin D through exposure to ten minutes of sunlight or intake of 200 IU daily (400 IU over age 50, 600 IU over age 70).

Another risk factor associated with osteoporosis in men is undiagnosed low levels of the sex hormone testosterone. Just as lack of estrogen leads to bone loss in women, the same holds true for testosterone in men. Blood testosterone levels can fall during long-term exercise, and resting levels may be lower in highly trained endurance athletes. It is possible that the male reproductive system may be blunted in response to endurance training.

Testosterone levels do decline naturally with age.

However, most men achieve greater peak bone mass levels than women and do not have the accelerated bone loss that women experience at menopause. It is possible that some men may not achieve peak bone density for genetic reasons, but also due to smoking and excess alcohol intake. Certain medications such as long-term glucocorticoid treatment may also adversely affect bone mass. Some men also develop osteoporosis for no identified reasons. ■

may not be able to meet calorie requirements solely from three meals daily. This can lead to weight loss or suboptimal recovery from daily training. Athletes may also be overwhelmed by the variety of foods offered in a dorm cafeteria and not feel confident that their food choices match their training requirements. They may not be familiar with the amount of carbohydrates they need to consume and feel uncertain of food preparation techniques and the fat content of certain items.

It is also possible to overeat at the dining hall where portions and choices are unlimited. Many athletes may also snack while studying and feel that they have fewer food restraints imposed upon them in terms of eating times and other limitations, and can feel somewhat out of control in regards to their food choices. Food may also be a large part of the social life at school, and excess calories can be consumed.

Eating in the dorm cafeteria can support a healthy sports diet with knowledge and planning. Athletes should appreciate what foods provide carbohydrates and balance these items with quality protein sources and healthy fats. For example, a grilled chicken breast can be consumed with rice, a steamed vegetable, and salad topped with olive oil. Athletes should understand that some fat can be consumed in the diet. It is a matter of balancing fat intake in the context of the day's food choices.

When eating in a dorm, it can also be very helpful to survey all the choices available at each meal and decide what foods to consume. Don't pile up on each dish or offering, but rather try to balance the meal by incorporating items from several food groups. Remember that the menu in the cafeteria is provided on a cycle. Your favorite foods and other interesting items will come around again. Treats can be part of the diet, as long as they are well-chosen items and in reasonable portions. It can be tempting to stay in the cafeteria and socialize with friends. However, this can lead to eating when you are not hungry and overeating.

For those athletes who cannot meet their nutritional requirements with the three daily meals offered, several options exist. Many cafeterias permit snacks such as sandwiches, fruit, or yogurt to be taken for consumption later. You can also keep a small fridge in your dorm room and stock fruit, yogurt, milk, cereal, and granola bars.

Snacks can also be purchased on campus between classes as your schedule permits. Fruit smoothies make excellent recovery snacks. Purchase your favorite sports drink if it will enhance your workouts and minimize fuel depletion, ultimately improving your recovery.

NUTRITION FOR COMPETITION

One of the ironies of swim training is that hours of preparation weekly culminates in a race or races lasting dozens of seconds to dozen of minutes. Another unique aspect of swim competition is the multiple number of heats and events in which a swimmer may compete over one to several days. International meets can last longer than one week. It is not unusual for a swimmer to compete in a heat in the morning and a final later that day or have several races scattered throughout the day. Travel to races is often required.

Before swimmers arrive at the start for competition, they likely have tapered their training for several days, resulting in the opportunity to increase muscle glycogen stores and arrive to competition race ready and fueled. Calorie needs may decrease somewhat or greatly depending on the extent of the taper, but a high percentage of the diet should come from carbohydrates so that the total grams of carbohydrates are optimal. The pre-competition meal should top off glycogen stores and increase blood glucose levels. Swimmers may have to very carefully time their meals throughout the competitive day in order to replenish stores after training and not overeat prior to the next race. Swimmers normally complete light warm-ups prior to competition and a swim-down after the event to improve recovery.

If carbohydrates must be consumed less than one hour prior to competition, emphasize 40–70 grams of a carbohydrate gel or liquid source such as a sports drink. For longer time spans such as two to four hours, larger and more solid carbohydrate foods can be consumed. Some tolerated choices include bagels, energy bars, fruit, crackers, and English muffins. Well-tolerated protein choices can augment this carbohydrate intake. Choices include lean turkey, yogurt, dairy and soy milk, and energy bars with a higher protein content. If traveling to competition,

The 40-30-30 Diet

A complicated low carbohydrate diet commonly referred to as the 40-30-30 diet gained popularity early on as the author of the book first outlining this diet claimed responsibility for the Olympic success of prominent collegiate swimmers. Some top competitors in triathlon also endorsed this diet and the sports nutrition products associated with the diet.

Despite the fact that this diet theory has been promoted for more than a decade, the benefits of this nutritional program for athletes continue to be anecdotal only, with no clinical studies measuring an improvement in athletic performance. Critics of the diet note that it hides a meal plan of less than 1,700 calories daily behind a complicated biochemical theory that includes hormonal pathways and promises of miraculous good health and disease prevention.

According to the theory, an athlete's diet should consist of 40 percent carbohydrates, 30 percent protein, and 30 percent fat, representing a sharp contrast to the recommended 60-15-25 breakdown advised to endurance athletes. It is contended that this lower consumption of carbohydrates, coupled with increased protein intake, allows the body to utilize more fat as an energy source by decreasing the production of insulin. In turn, this decreased production of insulin will suppress "bad" short-lived hormone-like compounds that increase inflammation in the body. In turn, "good" short-lived hormone production would be increased, and inflammation would be reduced.

The recommended nutrient percentages for endurance athletes are all relative to the amount of calories consumed. If a swimmer or another endurance athlete were to consume adequate calories for training, carbohydrate intake may or may not fall short of the amounts recommended. Over time, muscle glycogen would not be adequately replaced and training could be compromised. The nutrient that is exceptionally high in the 40-30-30 diet is protein. An athlete requiring 4,000 calories daily for endurance training would need to consume 400 grams of carbohydrate, which could fall short of adequately replacing muscle glycogen stores, and consume 300 grams of protein which greatly exceeds requirements.

Critics of the 40-30-30 plan also contend that the connection between insulin and these specific short-lived hormones is weak at best and not outlined in standard biochemistry texts, and that these hormones do not control all physiological functions in the body.

While future research may pinpoint scientifically measured techniques for increasing fat utilization during ultraendurance exercise, athletes should continue to train well on the nutrition guidelines currently recommend by sports nutritionists. ■

it is useful to bring some of your favorite and well-tolerated competition foods. Fluid considerations should be addressed throughout the competition. Swimmers may be in a warm and humid environment for several hours and should drink continuously. Urine should be pale in color if hydration levels are adequate.

DISTANCE SWIMMING

Long distance swimmers should start the race well fueled and adequately hydrated. A high carbohydrate intake can be combined with a taper several days prior to the race. High carbohydrate supplements can make this carbo-loading phase simpler. A high intake of fluid should be consumed leading up to the race. A pre-race meal can be consumed the morning of the swim. Liquid and easily digested foods high in carbohydrates will fill liver glycogen stores and raise blood glucose.

In events where there is an escort craft, feed on a pre-determined schedule during the race and prepare your feeds ahead of time. Practice drinking during longer swims. Swims longer than ninety minutes require carbohydrate replenishment. Aim for 60–75 grams per hour. Practice rolling on your back and drinking. Solid foods can be used when you tire of drinking. Try cut-up energy bars or gels. Aim to obtain feeds every twenty minutes. Set your watch to remind you to drink.

Be aware of the temperature during the race. Colder water temperatures burn fuel more quickly as you attempt to keep your body warm. Hot water feeds can be warming. In warmer water your fluid needs increase during competition. Try to keep hydrating fluids cool in warmer weather.

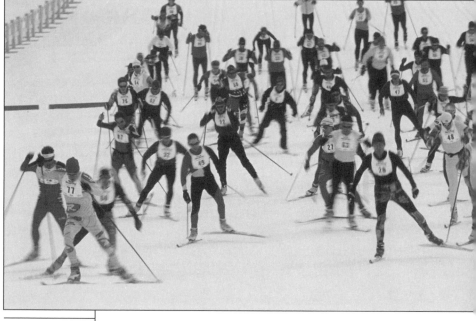

TOM MORAN PHOTO

chapter 13

NUTRITION FOR CROSS-COUNTRY SKIING

C ross-country skiing is one of the best endurance sports for improving your fitness level. This sport develops both upper and lower body strength, while stressing and enhancing both the aerobic and anaerobic energy systems. With origins in Scandinavia more than 4,000 years ago as a practical method of transportation, cross-country skiing is now part of high school and collegiate competition, and adult skiing at various levels. One-third of all Winter Olympic Games medals are awarded in cross-country skiing and related Nordic sports. Cross-country skiing is divided into two competitive styles. Classic or traditional skiing involves a straight-ahead gliding motion, and ski skating or freestyle incorporates a V-style glide and edge motion similar to in-line skating.

Just about anywhere that there are groomed trails and snow, there are organized cross-country ski competitions. Small race events may attract a few dozen local skiers, while the largest events attract more than 18,000 competitors and elite racers from foreign countries. Races can range in distance from one to several kilometers for the youngest competitors to 5K, 10K, 15K, and 20K races in collegiate and age-group racing. Endurance cross-country ski races can extend to 30K and more than 50K in distance. Some races may include relay teams. Elite racers may ski in endurance events from one hour to three hours or more depending on the length of the race. The rest of the pack may take twice to three times as long to finish the race. Training commitments can extend anywhere from seven to more than fifteen hours weekly, and vary with the level and competitive goals of the athlete.

Elite cross-country skiers are renowned for their astounding fitness as evidenced by their high VO_2 max, low levels of body fat, and low resting heart rates. Average daily energy expenditures for cross-country skiers are high. One study estimated that female skiers burned about 3,500 calories daily and men 5,000 calories daily when at the peak of training. Cross-country ski training consists of steady endurance, hill, and interval training. Of course, cross-country skiing also involves skill and technique. Calorie expenditure may diminish during specific times of the season when training incorporates off-season activities such as roller skiing, running, cycling, mountain biking, and weight training.

Cross-country skiers can benefit greatly from optimal endurance nutrition for recovery from the intense fuel demands of training. Endurance training also warrants fuel and fluid replacement during exercise. Proper nutrition also enhances the results of a resistance training program. Nutritional race preparation is very specific to the race distance and time in which the race is completed.

NUTRITION FOR TRAINING

Recovery Nutrition

Cross-country skiers should pay close attention to recovery nutrition, as their workouts often significantly deplete muscle glycogen stores. A full day of training followed by another demanding day requires that you replenish stores to ski at the desired level day after day. Elite skiers must meet their energy needs daily, while more recreational skiers or weekend warriors need to appreciate and balance the shifting fuel demands of their training program.

Skiers preparing for 50K or longer distances require high carbohydrate intakes ranging from 4.5 to 5.5 grams per pound of weight. A 140- or 165-pound skier would require at least 630 grams or 725 grams of carbohydrates respectively to recover from four to six hours of training. These longer training sessions necessitate adequate meal planning in order to consume the full carbohydrate amount. Emphasize concentrated sources of carbohydrates and sports nutrition supplements if required. Some of these carbohydrate calories can also be consumed during training in the form of bars, gels, and sports drinks. Training for distances between 20K and 50K also places demands on muscle glycogen stores. Skiers training for these distances require 3.0–4.5 grams carbohydrates per pound—more than 425 grams for the 140-pound skier and 600 grams for the 165-pound skier.

When training for shorter distances of less than 20K, carbohydrate requirements will not be as high. Sixty minutes of training, even at moderate to high intensity, demands about 2.25–3.0 grams per pound, or topping off at 400–500 grams daily of carbohydrate. High intensity interval training will deplete specific muscle fibers of glycogen, as will low intensity training lasting several hours. Recovery nutrition must be practiced after both these types of training sessions.

All skiers need to plan ahead regardless of their training program and competitive goals in order to begin the full recovery process. Strenuous workouts should followed within thirty minutes by 50–75 grams of carbohydrates, 24 ounces of fluid for every pound of weight lost during training, and small amounts of protein if desired. These choices allow the skier to rehydrate, replenish muscle glycogen stores, repair damaged muscle fibers, and support the immune system, all useful strategies after a good, hard workout in the cold weather.

Because of long endurance training sessions, protein may become a viable fuel source, supplying up to 15 percent of fuel usage toward the end of exercise. Skiers should consume the amounts of protein recommended for endurance athletes and aim for 0.5–0.8 grams per pound daily. Most skiers will meet their protein requirements with 70–110 grams for a 140-pound skier, and 85–130 grams for a 165-pound skier. Protein supplements are unnecessary, and these amounts can easily be met with a balanced and well-planned diet.

Keeping Your Immune System Healthy

As an endurance athlete you are mainly concerned with choosing the proper foods for maximizing energy and optimizing recovery. But you are probably aware that eating the right foods can also give your immune system a supportive boost and that your immune system may even be a bit fragile. Combining training with work and a personal life can overtax your resources, stress your body, and compromise your ability to fight infection. A strong immune system should result in fewer colds and viruses, and if you do get sick, recovery should be quicker. One thing serious athletes don't want to encounter is an unplanned halt to their training program due to illness. It is important for you to appreciate that specific foods can strengthen your immune system.

One of the first nutrients that may come to mind when you think about preventing colds is vitamin C, which has a widespread reputation as an immune system booster. While you may choose to supplement reasonably with this popular vitamin, don't minimize the importance of good food sources. Experts recommend a minimum of five servings of fruits and vegetables daily, but up to nine servings daily are ideal. Fruits and vegetables contain ample amounts of vitamin C, especially when superfresh. But fruits and vegetables also contain hundreds of phytochemicals that provide many preventative health benefits. Fruits and vegetables are also excellent sources of carotenoids such as beta-carotene, alpha-carotene, leutin, and lycopene, to name a few. Studies suggest that carotenoids may boost the activity of white blood cells called lymphocytes.

But the nutrients found in fruits

and vegetables are only one part of the immune system story. One downside of the low fat diet craze may be an inadequate intake of nutrients called essential fatty acids. Because your body cannot manufacture them, you need to ingest small amounts of linoleic acid and alpha-linolenic acid to support a strong immune system. Place an emphasis on alpha-linolenic acid, or omega-3 fatty acids. They are more limited in the North American diet and give your immune system a good boost. Good sources of these fatty acids include flax, canola, and walnut oils, soy milk, and soy nuts.

Minerals such as iron, zinc, and copper are also important in keeping your immune system healthy. Moderate amounts of these nutrients in your diet are entirely sufficient. In fact, an excess of these helpful nutrients may depress your immune system and exacerbate the infection process. But you can boost your immune system by ensuring your diet provides good food sources of these nutrients, and are unlikely to overdo them if you stick with good food sources and supplements providing only 100 percent of the Daily Values.

Another food that has intrigued researchers for its potential immune boosting properties is garlic. The immune boost in garlic probably comes from its most active ingredient called allicin. Research indicates that you may need the equivalent of one clove of garlic daily to receive its immunity-boosting benefits.

Good wholesome food sources can go a long way in keeping your immune system healthy. This means eating a variety of foods including plenty of fruits, vegetables, and whole grains. Taking a multivitamin-mineral supplement providing 100 percent of the daily values may also benefit your immune system.

(continued on page 276)

(continued from page 275)

Besides these helpful nutritional strategies for preventing illness, practice some other sensible health guidelines. Get plenty of sleep, avoid overtraining, and make sure rest is built into your program. Try to keep life stresses to a minimum and avoid individuals with colds whenever possible. Drinking carbohydrate beverages during and after exercise may also minimize the release of stress hormones brought on by hard training. Rapid weight loss also stresses the immune system, another good reason to practice the guidelines outlined in Chapter 7. ■

Fat should also comprise 20 to 25 percent of the total calories consumed. Though low body fat levels minimize the presence of "dead weight" for the skier, adequate fat is required to replenish muscle triglyceride stores depleted from prolonged training, and to provide essential fatty acids.

Off-Season

Calorie and carbohydrate requirements change as skiers alter their program with the change in seasons. Off season training, which may merely be designated by lack of snow, requires alternative forms of aerobic training, often in the forms of roller skiing, mountain biking, and running. Training volume and intensity may taper off during this time of year or be maintained through other competitive pursuits. Guidelines for carbohydrate intake based on training volume and intensity are provided in Chapter 4. After longer, low intensity training sessions, make sure to practice the principles of recovery nutrition within thirty minutes after exercise. Review seasonal changes in your training program and ascertain how your carbohydrate requirements may fluctuate depending on your off-season training.

Fluid and Food during Training

Consuming adequate fluids and carbohydrates during exercise is important for the skier year-round. Prepare for each training session by consuming plenty of water in the hours beforehand. Clear urine indicates that you are keeping up with your daily fluid needs. During training, even in colder weather, you can sweat as much as 2 quarts per hour if you are dressed warmly.

Cold weather exercise also results in fluid losses through exhalation. Dehydration can increase your risk of frostbite by decreasing blood flow to the extremities. But despite these fluid losses, carbohydrate replacement may be your top priority during cold weather. As reviewed in Chapter 5, sports drinks provide a balance between carbohydrates and fluid. You can even concentrate your drinks for a greater carbohydrate intake per ounce.

Replacing fluid losses in cold weather can be even more challenging than during hot weather when the drive to drink may be stronger. Cold weather can blunt your thirst, and the thought of a cold drink can make your teeth chatter. Hot decaffeinated tea mixed with plenty of honey can provide a carbohydrate boost. You can even dilute sweet drinks such as hot chocolate and hot apple cider for warming energy while training. These warm liquids provide several advantages. They are easier to drink when it is cold outside, provide a feeling of warmth, and increase blood flow to the extremities by dilating blood vessels. During cold weather exercise, aim for consuming at least one full 20-ounce water bottle per hour. Sports drinks can also be prepared with warm water.

Endurance training should be matched with 30–60 grams of carbohydrate consumption per hour. These carbohydrate amounts can be obtained from sports drinks (concentrated or regular strength), and gels and energy bars taken with water. Carbohydrate intake during exercise is especially important when pre-exercise eating is not optimal due to scheduling.

Nutrition for Weight Training

Weight training is an important component of many skiers' training programs and is especially useful for building the upper body strength required in cross-country skiing. As reviewed in Chapter 7, resistance training requires an additional 350–400 calories daily for the development of one pound of muscle mass. Consuming adequate calories when weight training makes adequate protein consumption relatively simple. Protein requirements of 0.5–0.7 grams per pound are easily met with quality protein sources in reasonable portions. More strenuous training sessions can receive a boost when you consume a sports drink during exercise to replenish fuel losses, particularly later in the training session.

Weight Management

While Olympic cross-country skiers are extremely lean when compared to the average male and female, ideal body fat levels are individual to the skier. Body fat contributes no strength advantage and must be carried, possibly limiting endurance and speed. Skiers should follow a balanced training program and a diet that supports optimal recovery from that program to arrive at a body composition that is good for their performance and health.

Losing body fat should be done carefully, and your diet should not be decreased by more than 200 to 300 calories daily. Weight loss efforts should occur well before high training loads and the important part of the competitive season arrives. To determine when your diet can be comfortably adjusted, keep a food journal for up to one week. Determine if there is any eating related to stress or boredom, rather than actual hunger, that can be reduced. Unnecessary fat and sugar can be reduced, as portions can be trimmed slightly for reasonable cutbacks in calories. Trying to lose weight too quickly can result in a loss of muscle mass and power, poor recovery, hormonal imbalances, and disordered eating.

Iron Status

Because of the heavy demands of training, cross-country skiers are a high-risk group for developing iron deficiency and anemia. Skiers complete a high volume of training and may train at altitude. Younger skiers need to meet both growth and exercise requirements, and female skiers need to replace losses from menstruation. Iron stores should be monitored regularly to prevent deficiency and anemia. Chapter 3 provides nutrition guidelines for increasing iron intake.

COMPETITION NUTRITION

Pre-exercise Eating

Whatever the length of the ski race that you will be completing, it is important that you are well fueled and physically and psychologically comfortable at the start line. For any event, a high carbohydrate and low fat meal is the optimal choice. The pre-race meal provides an opportunity for last-minute fueling to replenish liver and muscle glycogen stores and raise blood glucose levels. Skiers may also want to reduce the fiber content of their pre-competition meals to prevent any gastrointestinal distress on race day.

Shorter Events

Skiers competing in shorter events, such as 5K and 10K races performed at high intensity, should allow for adequate digestion time. Races with later start times may be preceded by a large breakfast and a lighter, high carbohydrate meal a few hours before the race. Small amounts of easily digested low fat protein can be incorporated into one of these meals. The pre-exercise meal should simply prevent hunger during the warm-up and race, leave the stomach feeling settled and the athlete satisfied, and maintain steady blood glucose levels. Hydrate well before a race, as dehydration can occur during your warm-up if you don't drink adequately beforehand. A sports drink may be a well-tolerated choice in the hour or two before the race and provides both carbohydrates and fluid. You can also emphasize warm drinks in the hour or two leading up to the race.

Longer Events

Preparation for events that will last longer than ninety minutes for the individual skier requires paying close attention to nutrition in the forty-eight hours or longer

Training in Cold Weather

Cross-country skiers spend a lot of time training and racing in cold weather. Just as hot weather requires sensible strategies for safe exercise, cold weather training also creates concerns for the endurance athlete. The inability to maintain a core temperature at or near 98.6 degrees Fahrenheit, or hypothermia, is the greatest risk posed by outdoor exercise in cold weather. When heat is drawn from the body faster than it can be replaced, the body cools. It then responds by restricting blood flow to the extremities. Some early warning signs of hypothermia include shivering and confusion. Risk of hypothermia can be aggravated when the weather changes quickly, on windy days, and when you become wet from sweat, rain, or snow.

Athletes can become acclimatized to cold weather, though this process is not as clearly understood as heat acclimatization and is also more difficult to attain. Some of the benefits that cold weather acclimatization can offer the athlete include increased blood flow to the extremities, elevated metabolic rate for increased generation of heat, and a slight increase in body fat. This higher metabolic rate also demands more calories from the athlete. Athletes with higher levels of body fat also have better cold tolerance than leaner athletes, as peripheral and core body temperatures tend to remain more stable. Very fit athletes also have a better tolerance to the cold. In addition to hypothermia, dehydration can also develop during cold weather exercise.

You don't stop sweating when exercising in the cold. A moderate rise in body temperature is accompanied by sweat, and overdressing for cold weather exercise also increases sweating. You also lose fluid when your respiratory tract warms and humidifies incoming cold and dry air. Offsetting these fluid losses and drinking in cold weather can be challenging—it is not always very appealing, and it may be hard to keep drinks from freezing. It may also not be convenient to carry and pull out fluids to drink in the cold weather.

Besides trying to keep up with your fluid needs, some nutritional strategies may help you beat the cold. When you train in cold weather you burn a greater amount of calories than you would in warmer weather. You still need to replenish carbohydrates to fuel your muscles and maintain high blood glucose levels. Cold weather causes you to use up muscle glycogen at a slightly higher rate, and shivering also uses carbohydrates for fuel. Just as in hot weather training, carbohydrates remain your number one fuel priority during endurance exercise.

Matching your fluid losses from cold weather training demands that you drink before you become thirsty. Put hot drinks in an insulated bottle. Keep the bottle close to your body if possible to keep it warm, or use a bladder hydration system designed for cold weather. Water alone is not likely to be adequate during cold weather exercise, as carbohydrate is needed to maintain blood glucose levels. You can use sports drinks mixed with warm water, hot apple cider, teas mixed with honey, or diluted hot cocoa.

Make sure you fuel up before a winter training session. Digestion revs up your body and produces heat. A high carbohydrate meal also tops off muscle glycogen stores and increases blood glucose levels. You can also keep cut-up energy bars stored close to your body to keep from freezing and stash a gel packet in a warm pocket for a nice glucose intake later during exercise. Set your watch to remind you to nibble and drink. ■

leading up to the event. For longer races exceeding 30K, the skier may choose to taper and fuel up on a high carbohydrate diet forty-eight to seventy-two hours before the event. Calorie needs may decrease somewhat prior to competition, but the skier should take in 4–5 grams of carbohydrates for every pound of weight to fully replenish and fill up muscle glycogen stores. Pay constant attention to hydration, and keep a water bottle with you at all times.

The night before the race consume a high carbohydrate meal. Some well-tolerated choices may include pasta, rice, potatoes, cooked vegetables (smaller amounts for some athletes), and breads. Emphasize lean proteins like poultry and fish. Stick with relatively bland and plain foods and avoid anything new, unusual, or spicy. Go easy on the fats, just enough to provide a bit of flavor.

The morning of the race, emphasize carbohydrates and small amounts of protein, and even fat that may improve cold tolerance and keep hunger at bay. Warm foods can be appealing before racing out in the cold. As in most endurance events, allowing three hours for digestion is adequate for most skiers, though those with sensitive stomachs may want to allow up to four hours. Aim for a pre-exercise meal providing more than 200 grams of carbohydrates. Use the carbohydrate food lists provided in Chapter 6 to plan an appropriate meal. Drink fluids up to the race. Warm fluids are fine, such as sports drinks mixed with warmer water or hot tea with honey.

During the Race

What you consume during endurance cross-country ski races is just as important as what you eat beforehand. Your carbohydrate reserves run low after seventy-five to ninety minutes, and consuming fluid and fuel during the race is essential.

Cold weather may dull your sense of thirst or make drinking less convenient, but pay close attention to fluid needs. Drink on a schedule and carry fluid with you. You may want to purchase a bladder system designed for skiers or carry an insulated water bottle around your waist. Choose a sports drink that provides a nice balance of fluid and carbohydrates. When glucose levels run low, a carbohydrate gel can provide a quick fix. Pay close attention to symptoms of bonking. Your concentration can decrease, you can feel cold and start to shiver, and you can feel hungry. Extra cold weather and high intensity efforts such as hill climbing may push up your carbohydrate requirements and increase your risk.

Skiers need to practice drinking during training so those skills are fine-tuned for race time. Start drinking fifteen minutes into the race as you settle into a rhythm. Skiing at a slight downhill, in the middle of the pack, or drafting off other skiers presents a good opportunity to drink. Try to slow down and drink at the feed stations provided. Bend the cup to form a spout and gulp fluid quickly. Some solid food items that may be provided include energy bars, cookies, brownies, and gels. Warming items may include soup and hot chocolate. Save the fluids you carry for consumption between feeds. Energy gels can be stashed away or taped somewhere to your clothing for a needed carbohydrate boost when fuel runs low.

Refueling after the race is also part of your race-day strategy. Consume plenty of liquids and 50–75 grams of carbohydrates within thirty minutes after finishing and again in several hours. This will improve your recovery and give you more energy to celebrate or begin preparation for the next race.

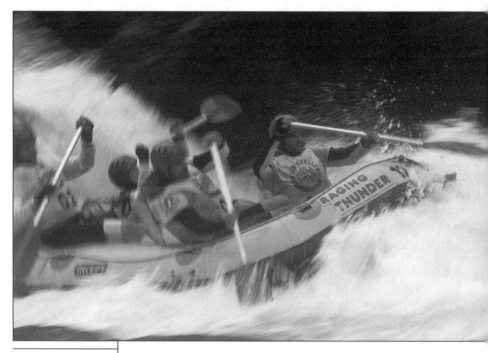

DAN CAMPBELL PHOTO

chapter 14

NUTRITION FOR ADVENTURE RACING

Adventure racing has been part of the New Zealand landscape for several decades, and the first official adventure race was founded in 1989. Since its inception, adventure racing has taken place all over the world, from Costa Rica to Tibet. Many North Americans are familiar with the Eco-Challenge that has been held in the U.S., Canada, and other parts of the world. These multiday races remain popular, but shorter and entry level adventure racing has also become popular, opening adventure racing to a greater field of competitors. Adventure racing now includes a multisport race with a team component, solo competitors, and races that vary greatly in length. Some popular adventure races include the Eco-Challenge, Raid Gauloises, Salomon X-Adventure Race Series, and Hi-Tec Adventure Races.

Races lasting longer than twenty-four hours may have several categories in order to allow more teams to complete the race. Longer races can also allow a support crew of one or two people to transport the team's gear to transition areas along the race course, while race personnel transport gear in "unsupported" races. Shorter or sprint races normally have a single transition area so that support team assistance is not required. Many races are designed to have a coed team, though this can vary among race categories.

Adventure races include a variety of sports such as mountain biking, trekking, mountaineering, navigation or orienteering, and rafting, canoeing, or kayaking.

Longer races may even include horseback riding, whitewater swimming, and caving. Some races have special tests that focus on team building and problem solving.

Adventure racing includes the following categories:

Expedition style races in which competitors take from three to ten days to complete a course covering 250–500 miles.

Stage races that last two days or longer, where competitors are timed while covering a specific distance. The team that wins has the shortest cumulative time over each day of racing.

Weekend races that cover 50–150 miles, with winning times between twelve and thirty hours.

Sprint races that include team and solo categories and which last from two to eight hours.

NUTRITION FOR TRAINING

Of course your training program will be determined by the makeup of the adventure race in which you will be competing. Adventure racing requires a good endurance and strength base and the necessary skills for the various sporting disciplines in which you will compete. Most adventure racers train for ten to twelve hours or more weekly, depending on the goal they have in mind, whether it is finishing or winning.

Endurance training adventure racers generally build an endurance base at 60 to 70 percent of maximum heart rate, and train for more than an hour at this intensity. Generally these workouts include cycling and/or running. Endurance training also consists of long hard workouts of back-to-back sports, such as hiking followed by canoeing, topped off with a bike or run. These workouts stress all areas of the body and help simulate an adventure race. You should practice carrying a pack and bring foods and fluids with you to simulate this aspect of the race. Adventure race training may include any or all of the following workouts:

- **Trekking**: Training for trekking consists of long, slow trail runs, fast hikes, and running and trekking sessions of two to three hours. Runs and hill work are incorporated into trekking sessions. In the winter, snowshoeing or cross-country skiing are great activities for maintaining an aerobic base. Indoor training on a treadmill or NordicTrack can also maintain your fitness.

- **Mountain biking**: Weekly sessions consist of road training for two to three hours and longer rides lasting up to five or six hours. Off-road skills can also be developed on a mountain bike.
- **Paddling:** Training for this section of the race also requires endurance training, as racing may require several hours of paddling. Training sessions should consist of two to three hours.
- **Strength training:** This may include two to three sessions weekly to build strength. Weekly sessions will cover the whole body.
- **Interval training:** These workouts can include running, hiking, or cycling hill repeats.

There are a wide variety of training modalities and distances associated with adventure racing. Endurance training is your main priority and requires that you focus on the following nutritional strategies during training:

Recovery nutrition: Endurance training requires that you begin the recovery process shortly after exercise. After training sessions lasting longer than ninety minutes, focus on consuming 0.5 grams of carbohydrates for every pound of weight. Consume 24 ounces of fluid for every pound of weight lost during exercise. Include sodium or salt in your post-exercise intake, particularly after training in the heat and humidity. Small amounts of protein can be added to the recovery snack. Of course recovery nutrition continues for the next twenty-four hours or until the next training session. Refer to Chapter 4 to ensure that your carbohydrate intake matches that day's training and recovery requirements. Round out your meals with adequate amounts of protein and fat.

Adequate fluid and food intake during training: Endurance training not only allows you to train your body for adventure racing, but also your gastrointestinal system and skills for eating and drinking during exercise. Practice consuming 4–8 ounces of fluid every fifteen to twenty minutes. Experiment to determine your favorite brands of sports drinks so that you can consume a variety of flavors while racing. Aim for 30–60 grams of carbohydrates per hour and up to 75–100 grams per hour for longer ultraendurance sessions. Experiment with a variety of carbohydrate sources such as gels and bars. During adventure racing you may also want to consume a variety of less conventional foods to relieve any taste boredom. Experiment with pretzels, granola bars, sugar candy, dried fruit, gorp, Pop Tarts, paninis, beef jerky, and anything that appeals to you and is well tolerated. Heavier foods can be consumed when lower intensity endurance training is the focus of that day's training. You can also bring along any "cooked" foods that you may be interested in consuming during the race such as instant soup and powdered mashed potatoes.

Practice nutrition guidelines for resistance training. Since strength training is an important part of your preparation for adventure racing, it is important that you practice the nutrition principles outlined in Chapter 7. If your goal is to build muscle mass, increase your calories by 350–400 daily above your current training requirements. Ensure that you obtain adequate protein in your diet and plenty of carbohydrates. Protein supplements are not required. During training you can consume a sports drink to provide carbohydrates to your muscles and enhance the quality of your exercise sessions. Recovery nutrition should also be practiced after an intense strength training session.

Practice eating while exercising. Since adventure racing is long and takes the whole day, day after day, learning to eat comfortably before or while exercising is essential. Practice eating as much as possible during training. Purposely run slowly, hike, or bike at a steady pace after eating. This will train your system to become accustomed to consuming food very close to exercise and allow you to determine your best tolerances and strategies to be used during racing. You will know what portions and foods to consume at varying intensities. Generally, during higher intensity sections of training, gels and liquid products work best, while solid foods are a welcome change at lower intensities.

COMPETITION NUTRITION

If you are traveling overseas to your adventure race, you may want to be careful about consuming local foods in exotic locations. Contracting a bacterial infection is a poor way to start the race. Bring some of your own items and practice good travel hygiene.

You should also consider carbohydrate loading before your day or week of racing. Rest for several days prior (you may be traveling) and consume a high percentage of carbohydrates in your diet. This will supercompensate your muscles with much needed glycogen. Shorter races lasting several hours require that you rest adequately and arrive well fueled and adequately hydrated, but carbohydrate loading is not required.

While carbohydrates should predominate, you also require a mix of protein and fat during the race. During more intense races, you will burn several thousand calories daily. Aim to consume 300–400 calories per hour to replaces losses. Every racer has his or her own personal tolerances, but aim for the maximum that your body can handle. You are still likely to maintain a caloric deficit over the course of the race even with your best efforts.

As in most endurance competitions, you need to maintain a high carbohydrate intake to maintain blood glucose levels and supply your muscles with fuel. Your body should provide enough stored fat for your endurance efforts. Aim for 50–100 grams of carbohydrates per hour while exercising. You can also consume small amounts of proteins as tolerated when refueling during long races.

Carrying your food and fluid with you is a key component of adventure racing. Foods that are light in weight, calorically dense, low volume, appealing, and non-melting or nonperishable are likely to work best. Of course carry your favorite energy bars or gels, meal replacements, and some real foods. Real foods include trail mix, candy such as gummy bears, fruit roll-ups, dried fruit, and beef and turkey jerky. Some racers may even carry heavier items such as a sandwich or burrito, which can be carried early on in that segment of the race to lighten your load. You can even

Do Nutritional Needs Differ for Males and Females?

For the past several years, researchers have become increasingly aware that much of the data on exercise physiology, muscle metabolism, and nutrition has been conducted mainly on male participants. For years it has been assumed that these scientific results can be generalized to female athletes. Fortunately, in the past decade researchers have begun to investigate potential gender differences regarding nutritional requirements for exercise.

The nutritional implications of gender differences may be especially important for ultraendurance exercise such as adventure racing, long distance running, and long distance swimming. It appears that women burn a high amount of fat and a lower amount of carbohydrates at a given intensity, and theories abound that females can outperform males in ultraendurance events. A study conducted in South Africa compared equally trained male and female distance runners over 42K and 90K distances. At the 42K distance, the females performed equally to the males. But at the 90K mark the female athletes sustained a greater fraction of their VO_2 max. There are well-established differences between male and female athletes. The average male has large muscle mass, lower body fat, and a greater aerobic capacity, and is likely to outpower female athletes in strength events.

Several years ago, one study raised the question of whether carbohydrate loading could actually increase muscle glycogen stores in female athletes. A later study by the same group determined that when energy intake was equal between males and females, and the appropriate number of grams of carbohydrate per pound of weight was provided, that both groups similarly increased muscle glycogen stores.

The same type of study was also completed on recovery nutrition. Whether athletes were provided a carbohydrate-only solution or a mix of carbohydrate and protein, both males and females resynthesized glycogen adequately. It also appears that women benefit from the same guidelines as men regarding carbohydrate consumption during exercise. Another study has determined that there were no real

differences between men and women in the amount and manner in which carbohydrates were utilized during exercise.

One area of concern for female athletes may be the issue of body fat. There have been a greater number of female athletes reaching lower body fat levels that are comparable to those seen in male athletes. But data suggests that women are more prone to defend or maintain body weight than men. However, many experts are concerned that female athletes who strive for excess leanness may experience hormonal imbalances, nutrient deficiencies, and early osteoporosis and fractures. ■

rehydrate items such as mashed potatoes, powdered milk, and stuffing that have been placed in Ziploc plastic bags. You can also organize your foods for several days of racing. Each day's menu can be placed in large Ziploc plastic bags and then labeled properly. This way the appropriate bag can be obtained at the transition area.

Bottled water is essential. You should also carry water purification tablets to treat water found along the course. Powdered sports drinks can be reconstituted. Fluid can be conveniently carried in a bladder hydration system. You can also experiment with waist belts or water bottle holsters that attach to your backpack. Determine how much water you will need to carry with you during the race, depending on the length of the race and the placing of transition areas. Aim to drink 20–24 ounces per hour, or 6–7 quarts daily. Salty foods should also be carried, as well as salt packets and salt tablets. Remember to drink on a schedule. A carbohydrate-containing drink also fuels your brain and provides sodium. Keep in mind that dehydration can increase your risk for developing both hyperthermia and hypothermia. Also keep in mind that it is best to prevent dehydration. Drink before you are thirsty. Other signs of dehydration include headache, loss of appetite, infrequent urination, rapid heart rate, shortness of breath, and fatigue.

Eat on a schedule as well. Know what your total food consumption should be for that day. Try to plan the best times to eat based on the activity and terrain. Save your liquid carbohydrates for higher intensity endeavors and solid foods for when the intensity slows up a bit. Protein foods that may be appealing and eaten on the run include string cheese, peanuts, peanut butter, and canned tuna. Plan to eat every thirty to sixty minutes, and set a watch to remind teammates (you are only as fast as your slowest teammate) to eat. Keep food readily accessible in pockets and waistbands so that the effort of obtaining food is not too great. Practice consuming small, consistent amounts throughout the race.

For longer races that allow a support crew, many calories can be consumed in the transition area and this is your chance to replenish. Your crew can provide you with a substantial meal while you prepare for the next event. Some items consumed may include burritos, stew, grilled cheese, rice, meat, and pasta. Liquid meal replacements that provide more than 300 calories can also be consumed with the meal. You can also rely on dehydrated meals. Unsupported races require that you plan your transition meals carefully and have items ready for consumption in your gear. During shorter races, competitors may transition and load up on carbohydrates from easy items such as concentrated drinks and gels.

APPENDIXES

APPENDIX A: GLYCEMIC INDEX OF FOODS

High Glycemic Foods	(GI > 70)
Maltodexrin	105
Dates	103
Parsnips	97
French baguette	95
Rice, instant	90
Rice Chex	89
Potato, baked	85
Corn Chex	83
Corn Flakes	83
Rice Krispies	82
Pretzels	81
Wheat bread	78
Donut	76
Total cereal	76
Waffle	76
Cheerios	74
Graham wafers	74
Puffed wheat	74
Kaiser roll	73
Bagel, white	72
Watermelon	72
Bread, white	71
Millet	71
Cream of wheat	70
Melba toast	70
Potato, mashed	70

Moderate Glycemic Foods	(GI 50–69)	Low Glycemic Foods	(GI < 50)
Shredded Wheat	69	Porridge oatmeal	49
Cake, angel food	67	Bulgar	48
Croissant	67	Grapefruit juice	48
Pineapple	66	Mixed grain bread	48
Couscous	65	Oat bran bread	48
High fiber rye crispbread	65	Grapes	47
Oat kernel bread	65	Peach	47
Black bean soup	64	Lactose	46
Raisins	64	Orange	44
Muffin	62	Lentil soup	44
Ice cream	61	All Bran	42
Pizza, cheese	60	Apple juice	41
Apricots	57	Apple	38
Pita bread, white	57	Lentils	38
Mango	56	Navy beans	38
Muesli	56	Kidney beans	37
Buckwheat	55	Pear	37
Oat bran	55	Spaghetti, wholemeal	37
Rice, brown	55	Rye	34
Spaghetti, durum	55	Chickpeas	33
Sweet corn	55	Yogurt, fruited	33
Banana	54	Fettucine	32
Cake, pound	54	Milk, skim	32
Sweet potato	54	Barley	25
Orange juice	52	Fructose	22
Barley, cracked	50		

APPENDIX B: FACTS ABOUT VITAMINS

VITAMINS	DRI	MAJOR SOURCE	MAJOR FUNCTIONS
Water-soluble	**RDA for Ages 31–50**		
Thiamin (vitamin B_1)	Males: 1.2 mg/day Females: 1.1 mg/day	Wheat germ, whole grain breads and cereal, organ meats, lean meats, legumes	Energy production from carbohydrates, essential for healthy nervous system
Riboflavin (vitamin B_2)	Males: 1.3 mg/day Females: 1.1 mg/day	Milk and dairy products, green leafy vegetables, lean meats, beans	Energy production from carbohydrates and fats, healthy skin
Niacin (nicotinamide, nicotinic acid)	Males: 16 mg/day Females: 14 mg/day	Lean meats, fish, poultry, whole grains, peanuts	Energy production from carbohydrates, synthesis fat, blocks release FFA
Vitamin B_6 (pyridoxine)	Males: 1.3 mg/day > 51 yr.: 1.7 mg/day > 70 yr.: 1.7 mg/day Females: 1.3 mg/day > 51 yr.: 1.5 mg/day > 70 yr.: 1.5 mg/day	Liver, lean meats, fish, poultry, legumes, bran cereal	Role in protein metabolism, necessary for formation hemoglobin and red blood cells, synthesis essential fatty acids, required for glycogen breakdown
Vitamin B_{12} (cobalamin)	Males: 2.4 mcg/day Females: 2.4 mcg/day	Lean meats, poultry, dairy products, eggs	Formation of red blood cells, metabolism nervous tissue, involved folate metabolism, formation DNA
Biotin	Males: 30 mcg/day Females: 30 mcg/day	Meats, legumes, milk, egg yolk, whole grains	Role in metabolism of carbohydrates, protein, fat

VITAMINS	DRI	MAJOR SOURCE	MAJOR FUNCTIONS
Water-soluble	**RDA for Ages 31–50**		
Pantothenic acid	Males: 5 mg/day Females: 5 mg/day	Liver, lean meats, eggs, salmon, all animal and plant foods	Role in metabolism carbohydrates, protein, fat
Vitamin C	Males: 90 mg Females: 75 mg	Citrus fruits, green leafy vegetables, broccoli, peppers, strawberries, potatoes	Essential for connective tissue development, role in iron absorption, antioxidant, wound healing
Fat-soluble	**RDA**		
Vitamin A (retinol, provitamin carotenoids)	Males: 900 mcg Females: 700 mcg	Liver, milk, cheese, fortified margarine, Carotenoids in plant foods orange, red, deep green in color	Maintains healthy tissue in skin and mucous membranes, essential night vision, bone development
Vitamin D (cholecalciferol)	Males: 200 IU/day Females: 200 IU/day Males: > 51 yr.: 400 IU > 70 yr.: 600 IU Females: > 51 yr.: 400 IU > 70 yr.: 600 IU	Vitamin D fortified milk and margarine, fish oil, action of sunlight on skin	Increases intestinal absorption of calcium, promotes bone and tooth formation
Vitamin K (phylloquinone)	Males: 120 mcg Females: 90 mcg	Liver, soybean oil, spinach, cauliflower, green leafy vegetables	Essential normal blood clotting

APPENDIX B: FACTS ABOUT MINERALS

MINERALS	DRI	MAJOR SOURCE	MAJOR FUNCTIONS
Major Minerals	**RDA for Ages 31–50**		
Calcium	Males: 1,000 mg Females: 1,000 mg Males: >50 yr.: 1,200 mg > 70 yr.: 1,200 mg Females: > 50 yr.: 1200 mg > 70 yr.: 1200 mg	Milk, cheese, yogurt, ice cream, dried peas and beans, dark green leafy vegetables	Bone formation, enzyme activation, nerve impulse transmission, muscle contraction
Phosphorus	Males: 700 mg Females: 700 mg	Protein foods: meat, poultry, fish, eggs, milk, cheese, dried peas and beans, whole grains	Bone formation, cell membrane structure, B vitamin activation, component of ATP-CP, and other important organic compounds
Magnesium	Males: 420 mg Females: 320 mg	Milk, yogurt, dried beans, nuts, whole grains, tofu, green vegetables, chocolate	Roles in protein synthesis, glucose metabolism, muscle contraction
Trace Minerals	**RDA for Ages 31–50**		
Iron	Males: 8 mg Females: 18 mg > 50 yr.: 8 mg	Organ meats, lean meats, poultry, shellfish, dried peas and beans, whole grain products, green leafy vegetables	Hemoglobin formation, oxygen transport
Zinc	Males: 11 mg Females: 8 mg	Organ meats, meat, fish, poultry, shellfish, nuts, whole grain products	Part of enzymes involved in energy metabolism, immune function

B

MINERALS	DRI	MAJOR SOURCE	MAJOR FUNCTIONS
Trace Minerals	**RDA for Ages 31–50**		
Copper	Males: 900 mcg Females: 900 mcg	Organ meats, meat, fish, poultry, shellfish, nuts, bran cereal	Role in use of iron and hemoglobin by body, involved in connective tissue formation and oxidation
Fluoride	Adequate intake Males: 4 mg Females: 3 mg	Milk, egg yolks, drinking water, seafood	Helps form teeth and bones
Selenium	Males: 70 mcg Females: 55 mcg	Meat, fish, poultry, organ meats, seafood, whole grains and nuts from selenium-rich soil	Part of antioxidant enzyme
Chromium	Adequate intake Males: 35 mcg Females: 25 mcg	Organ meats, meats, oysters, cheese, whole grain products, beer	Enhances insulin function as glucose tolerance factor
Iodine	Males: 150 mcg Females: 150 mcg	Iodized table salt, seafood, water	Part of thyroxine, which plays role in reactions involving cellular energy
Manganese	Adequate intake Males: 2.3 mg Females: 1.8 mg	Beet greens, whole grains, nuts, legumes	Part of essential enzyme systems
Molybdenum	Males: 45 mcg Females: 45 mcg	Legumes, cereal grains, dark green leafy vegetables	Part of essential enzymes involved in carbohydrate and fat metabolism

▪
APPENDIX C: COMPARISON OF SPORTS NUTRITION PRODUCTS

COMMERCIAL SPORTS DRINKS (8 OZ. SERVING)					
Product	Type of Carbohydrate	Carbohydrate Concentration	Calories	Carbohydrate (grams)	Sodium (milligrams)
Accelerade	Sucrose, fructose, maltodextrin (also contains small amounts branched chain amino acids)	7.75%	93	17	127.0
All Sport	Fructose, sucrose	7%	70	19	55.0
Body Fuel	Maltodextrin, fructose	7%	70	17	70.0
Coca-Cola	High fructose corn syrup, sucrose	12%	108	29	9.0
Cytomax	Fructose, maltodextrin, polylactate, glucose	8%	83	19	70.0
Endura	Glucose polymers, fructose	6%	60	15	92.0
Exceed	Glucose polymer, fructose	7%	70	17	50.0
Gatorade	Sucrose, glucose	6%	50	14	110.0
Gookinaid	Glucose, fructose	5%	43	10	69.0
Hydra Fuel	Glucose polymer, fructose, glucose	7%	66	16	25.0
Met-Rx ORS	Rice syrup solids, glucose	8%	70	19	125.0
Orange Juice	Fructose, sucrose	11–15%	112	26	2.7
Perform	Glucose, fructose, maltodextrins	7%	60	16	110.0
Performance	Maltodextrin, fructose	10%	100	25	115.0
PR Solution	Maltodextrin, fructose	12.5%	120	30	50.0
Powerade	Fructose, sucrose	6%	55	14	50.0
Red Bull	Sucrose, glucose	12%	112	28	215.0

C

COMMERCIAL SPORTS DRINKS (8 OZ. SERVING)

Product	Type of Carbohydrate	Carbohydrate Concentration	Calories	Carbohydrate (grams)	Sodium (milligrams)
Revenge	Maltoxdextrin, fructose	4.2%	50	10	48.0
Ultima	Maltodextrin	1.7%	16	4	8.0
Warp Aide	Fructose, maltodextrin	8%	70	19	80.0
Water		0%	0	0	0.0

RECOVERY DRINKS

Product	Serving Size	Calories	Carbohydrate	Protein	Fat
Boost	8 oz. can	240	33	15	6.0
EnduroxR4	2 scoops	280	53	14	1.5
Ensure	8 ounce can	250	40	9	6.0
Gatorlode	2 scoops	200	49	0	0.0
GatorPro	11 oz. can	360	59	17	6.0
Metabolol	2 scoops	200	24	14	5.0
Metabolol II	2 scoops	260	40	18	3.0
Met-Rx	1 packet	260	24	37	2.0
Optimizer	2 scoops	280	58	11	0.0
Physique	4 scoops	210	38	14	0.0
UltraFuel	16 oz.	400	100	0	0.0

CARBOHYDRATE GELS

Product	Serving	Calories	Carbohydrate	Sodium
Clif Shot	32 g packet (1.1 oz.)	100	37	50
GU	32 g packet (1.1 oz.)	100	30	20
PowerGel	41 g packet (1.1 oz.)	110	33	50

APPENDIX D: SAMPLE MENUS

Sample menus of varying calorie and carbohydrate levels are provided here. You can adjust portions and make substitutions as desired to raise or lower calorie and carbohydrate intake. The vegetarian menus can also be used by animal protein eaters to obtain additional meal ideas, and vegetarians can utilize the animal protein-containing menus and make plant protein substitutions as desired. All menus were calculated utilizing the Nutritionist III software program.

2,200 calories 300 g carbohydrate 140 g protein 63 g fat	2,200 calories 510 g carbohydrate 120 g protein 63 g fat	2,400 calories 330 g carbohydrate 122 g protein 73 g fat
Grain cereal, cooked, 1 cup Banana, 1 large Cottage cheese, 1/2 cup Nuts, 1 Tbsp.	Orange juice, 1 cup French Toast, 2 slices Strawberries, 1 cup	Oatmeal, cooked, 1 cup Apple, 1 medium Juice, 8 oz.
Recovery smoothie: Dairy milk, 12 oz. Frozen fruit, 1 cup Granola, low fat, 1/2 cup	Low fat cheese, 2 oz. Bread, 2 slices Tomato, 1 whole Yogurt with fruit, 1 cup Pear, 1 whole	Soy milk, 8 oz. Strawberries, 1 cup Chicken, 3 oz. Whole grain bread, 2 slices Pretzels, 1 1/2 oz.
Tuna salad, low fat, 3 oz. Bread, 2 slices Lentil salad, 1/2 cup Juice, 8 oz.	Crackers, 8 small Hummus, 1/2 cup Carrots, 3 Avocado, 1/4 whole	Bagel, 4 oz. Peanut butter, 2 tsp. Pear, 1 large
Salmon, 6 oz. Buckwheat, cooked, 1 cup Asparagus, 1 cup Salad, 2 cups Olive oil, 2 tsp. Salad dressing, 2 Tbsp.	Rice, cooked, 1 1/2 cups Shrimp, cooked, 6 oz. Red pepper, 1 whole Broccoli, cooked, 1 cup Sesame seed oil, 1 Tbsp.	Beef strips, 3 oz. Noodles, cooked, 2 cups Bread, 1 slice Olive oil, 2 tsp. Mixed vegetables, 1 cup
Sorbet, 1/2 cup Peach, 1 medium	Mango, 1 whole Papaya, 1 cup	

D

2,400 calories 382 g carbohydrate 85 g protein 68 g fat	2,800 calories, 439 g carbohydrate 132 g protein 69 g fat	2,800 calories 440 g carbohydrate 145 g protein 64 g fat
English muffin, 1 whole Cream cheese, 2 Tbsp. Jam, 2 Tbsp. Grapefruit juice, 12 oz. Egg, 1 whole	Muesli, 3/4 cup Apple, 1 medium Raisins, 3 Tbsp. Soy milk, 1 cup Almonds, 6 nuts	Oatmeal, cooked, 1 1/2 cups Skim milk, 8 oz. Wheat germ, 4 Tbsp. Bread, 2 slices Jam, 2 Tbsp. Orange juice, 8 oz.

Pinto beans, 1/2 cup
Rice, cooked, 1 cup
Tortilla, 1 whole
Salsa, 4 Tbsp.
Cheese, 1 oz.
Avocado, 1/8 whole
	Energy bar, 1 medium
	Juice, 8 oz.
	
	Chicken tacos:
	  Chicken, 3 oz.
	  Beans, 1/2 cup
	  Rice, cooked, 2/3 cup
	  Tortillas, 2 large
	  Oil, 2 tsp.
		Chicken, 4 oz.
		Mayonnaise, light, 2 Tbsp.
		Rice and bean salad,
		  1 cup
		Grapes, 1 cup

Granola bar, 1 Peaches, 2 Almonds, 1 Tbsp.	Papaya, 1 whole Crackers, 2 oz. Cream cheese, 2 Tbsp.	Energy bar, 1 Banana, 1 Yogurt with fruit, 1

Pasta, cooked, 2 cups
Lean beef, 3 oz.
Marinara sauce, 1 cup
Green salad, 2 cups
Salad dressing, 2 Tbsp.
	Risotto:
	  Beef, 4 oz.
	  Broccoli, 1 cup
	  Rice, cooked, 2/3 cup
	  Bread, 2 slices
	  Oil, 2 tsp.
		Tofu, 6 oz.
		Soba noodles, cooked,
		  2 cups
		Vegetables, 2 cups
		Sesame seed oil, 3 Tbsp.

Frozen Yogurt, 1 cup Blueberries, 1/2 cup		

APPENDIX D: SAMPLE MENUS

3,200 calories	3,300 calories	3,600 calories
500 g carbohydrate	520 g carbohydrate	635 g carbohydrate
158 g protein	137 g protein	136 g protein
70 g fat	90 g fat	68 g fat

Bread, 2 slices	Waffles, 4 squares	Raisin bran, 1 1/2 cups
Peanut butter, 1 Tbsp.	Syrup, 1/2 cup	Milk, 8 oz.
Citrus juice, 12 oz.	Berries, 1 cup	Grapefruit, 1 whole
Banana, 1 whole	Hard boiled egg, 1	Bagel, 3 oz.
Yogurt, plain, 1 cup	Soy milk, 12 oz.	Cheese, low fat, 2 oz.
Tuna, 4 oz.	Roast turkey, 3 oz.	Recovery drink, 16 oz.
Mayonnaise, 1 Tbsp.	Avocado spread, 4 Tbsp.	Juice, 8 oz.
Pita bread, 1 round	Pita, toasted, 1 round	Banana, 1 large
Pretzels, 1 1/2 oz.	Plums, 3 medium	
Raw vegetable salad,	Juice, 12 oz.	Peanut butter, 1 Tbsp.
1 cup	Yogurt, nonfat, 8 oz.	Jam, 2 Tbsp.
		Bread, 2 slices
Soy milk, 12 oz.	Pasta, cooked, 3 cups	Orange, 1 medium
Peach slices, 1 cup	Marinara sauce,	Yogurt with fruit, 8 oz.
Granola, low fat, 1/4 cup	1 1/2 cups	
	Lean beef, 3 oz.	Grilled chicken, 6 oz.
Halibut, 8 oz.	Bread, 2 slices	Sweet potatoes, 1 large
Millet, cooked, 1 cup	Salad, 2 cups	Peas, cooked, 1 cup
Asparagus, 1 cup	Olive oil, 3 tsp.	Bread, 2 slices
Flaxseed oil, 2 tsp.	Salad dressing, 2 Tbsp.	Olive oil, 5 tsp.
		Fruit salad, 1 cup
Sorbet, 1 1/2 cup		
Fig cookies, 2 whole		

D

3,600 calories
640 g carbohydrate
110 g protein
70 g fat

Grits, cooked, 1 cup
Raisins, 2 Tbsp.
Yogurt, nonfat, plain, 1 cup
Cherries, 20
Cashews, 1 Tbsp.

Hummus, 1/2 cup
Pita bread, 2 rounds
Celery, pepper, carrots,
  2 cups
Apple juice, 12 oz.

Bagel, 4 oz.
Nut butter, 2 Tbsp.
Apple, 1 large

Pork tenderloin, 4 oz.
Rice, cooked, 1 1/2 cups
Corn, 1/2 cup
Mushrooms, 1/4 cup
Bread, 2 slices
Olive oil, 4 tsp.

Sherbert, 1 cup
Raspberries, 1 cup

4,000 calories
600 g carbohydrate
180 g protein
105 g fat

Bran flakes, 1 cup
Milk, 1 cup
English muffin, 2
Cheese, melted,
  low fat, 2 oz.
Smoothie:
  Soy milk, 12 oz.
  Banana, 1
  Wheat germ, 3 Tbsp.

Sports Drink, 40 oz.

Beef and bean burritos:
  Beef, 8 oz.
  Rice, cooked, 1/5 cup
  Beans, 1 cup
  Tortillas, 2 large
  Salsa, 1 cup
  Canola oil, 4 tsp.

Gingersnaps, 6
Juice, 8 oz.

Tofu stir-fry:
  Tofu, 4 oz.
  Brown rice, cooked,
    1 1/2 cups
  Sweet peppers, cooked,
    1 cup
  Broccoli, cooked, 1 cup

Granola bar, 1
Sorbet, 2 cups
Figs, 3

4,300 calories
760 g carbohydrate
140 g protein
87 g fat

Pancakes, 4 small
Maple syrup, 3/4 cup
Banana, 1 large
Raisins, 2 Tbsp.
Nuts, 1 Tbsp.
Soy milk, 12 oz.

Sports Drink, 40 oz.

Burrito:
  Chicken, 5 oz.
  Rice, cooked, 2 cups
  Pinto beans, 1 cup
  Avocado, 1/4 whole
  Salsa, 1/2 cup

Linguine, cooked, 3 cups
Mixed vegetables, 1 cup
Bread, 2 slices
Olive oil, 2 Tbsp.
Salad, 2 cups
Salad dressing, 2 Tbsp.

Frozen yogurt, 2 cup
Cookies, 2
Strawberries, 1 cup

APPENDIX D: SAMPLE MENUS—VEGETARIAN

2,200 calories 370 g carbohydrate 90 g protein 50 g fat	2,400 calories 400 g carbohydrate 90 g protein 54 g fat	2,800 calories 470 g carbohydrate 110 g protein 64 g fat
Farina, cooked, 1 cup Skim milk, 8 oz. Brazil nuts, 1 Tbsp. Apple, 1 Orange juice, 12 oz.	Muesli, 1/2 cup Soy or dairy yogurt, 8 oz. Blueberries, 1 cup	Waffles, 2 small Maple syrup, 4 oz. Raspberries, 1 cup Skim milk, 1 cup
Soy burger, 1 patty Bun, 1 whole Cheese, low fat, 1 oz. Lentil salad, 1/2 cup Vegetables, raw, 1 cup Avocado, 1/8 whole	Garbanzo beans, 1/3 cup Salad with greens and vegetables, 3 cups Roll, 1 large Cheese, low fat, 2 oz. Grapefruit juice, 8 oz.	Hummus, 1/2 cup Rice, cooked, 1/2 cup Lentil salad, 1/2 cup Pita bread, 1 round Carrots and celery, 2 cups
Kidney beans, 1 cup Rice, cooked, 1 cup Tortilla, 1 whole Green salad, 1 cup Salad dressing, 2 Tbsp.	Energy bar, 1 medium Apple, 1 Tempeh, 1/2 cup Rice, 1 1/4 cups cooked Broccoli, cooked, 1 cup Sesame seed oil, 1 Tbsp.	Bagel, 4 oz. Cheese, low fat, 2 oz. Apple, 1 Tofu, 4 oz. Soba noodles, cooked, 2 cups Greens, cooked, 1 cup Sesame seed oil, 1 Tbsp.
Granola bar, 1 whole Peach, 1 whole Yogurt with fruit, 8 oz.		Pear, 1 large

D

3,200 calories
570 g carbohydrate
103 g protein
64 g fat

Pancakes, 4 small
Syrup, 6 Tbsp.
Raisins, 2 Tbsp.
Apple juice, 8 oz.

Soy or dairy yogurt
  with fruit, 8 oz.
Almonds, 2 Tbsp.

Bean soup, 1 1/2 cups
Rye crackers, 4
Vegetable salad, 1 cup
Soy milk, 12 oz.

Potato, 1 large
Kidney beans, 1 cup
Cheese, low fat, 1 oz.
Green salad, 2 cups
Salad dressing, 3 Tbsp.

Frozen yogurt, 1 cup
Mango, 1 large

3,600 calories
600 g carbohydrate
133 g protein
96 g fat

Bran flakes, 1 1/2 cups
Wheat germ, 2 Tbsp.
Soy or dairy milk, 8 oz.
Peach, 1 medium

Recovery Drink:
Juice, 12 oz.
Yogurt, 1 cup
Banana, 1 whole

Nut butter, 2 Tbsp.
Bread, 2 slices
Bean soup, 1 cup
Raw vegetables, 1 cup

Tofu, 8 oz.
Peas, 1 cup
Noodles, 2 cups
Rolls, 2
Vegetable oil, 2 Tbsp.
Green Salad, 2 cups
Salad dressing, 2 Tbsp.

Sports drink, 40 oz.

4,000 calories
685 g carbohydrate
128 g protein
102 g fat

Oatmeal, cooked,
  1 1/2 cups
Skim milk, 1 cup
Wheat germ, 2 Tbsp.
Orange juice, 12 oz.
Yogurt, 1 cup
Apple, 1 large

Sports Drink, 40 oz.

Thin crust pizza,
  easy cheese, 3 slices
Green salad, 2 cups
Salad dressing, 2 Tbsp.
Soy milk, 8 oz.

Pretzels, 2 oz.
Hummus, 1/2 cup
Raw vegetables, 1 cup

Spaghetti, cooked, 3 cups
Marinara sauce, 2 cups
Parmesan cheese, 3 Tbsp.
Italian bread, 2 slices
Olive oil, 1 Tbsp.

Sorbet, 2 cups
Fig bars, 3

BIBLIOGRAPHY

Armstrong, Lawrence E. 2000. *Performing in Extreme Environments.* Champaign, IL: Human Kinetics.

———. 2002. Caffeine, body fluid–electrolyte balance, and exercise performance. *International Journal of Sport Nutrition and Exercise Metabolism* 12 (2): 189–206.

Ball, T., et al. 1995. Periodic carbohydrate replacement during 50 minutes of high intensity cycling improves subsequent sprint performance. *International Journal of Sport Nutrition* 5: 151–158.

Beal, K. and M. Manore. 1994. The prevalence and consequences of subclinical eating disorders in female athletes. *International Journal of Sports Nutrition* 4: 175–195.

Below, P., et al. 1995. Fluid and carbohydrate ingestion independently improve performance during 1 hour intense exercise. *Medicine and Science in Sports and Exercise* 27: 200–210.

Benson, J., et al. 1996. Nutritional aspects of amenorrhea in the female athlete triad. *International Journal of Sport Nutrition* 6: 134–145.

Berning, J. 1996. The role of medium chain triglycerides in exercise. *International Journal of Sport Nutrition* 6: 121–133.

Blom, T., et al. 1987. The effects of different post-exercise sugar diets on the rate of muscle glycogen resynthesis. *Medicine and Science in Sports and Exercise* 19: 491–496.

Brand-Miller, Jennie, et al. 1999. *The Glucose Revolution.* New York: Marlowe and Company.

Brooks, G., et al. 1991. Increased dependence on blood glucose after acclimatization to 4,300 meters. *Journal of Applied Physiology* 70 (2): 919–927.

Brown, G., et al. 2000. Effect of anabolic precursors on serum testosterone concentrations and adaptations to resistance training in young men. *International Journal of Sport Nutrition and Exercise Metabolism* 10: 340–359.

Burke, L., et al. 1993. Muscle glycogen storage after prolonged exercise: Effect of the glycemic index of carbohydrate feedings. *Journal of Applied Physiology* 75: 1019–1023.

———. 1996. Muscle glycogen storage after prolonged exercise: Effect of the frequency of carbohydrate feedings. *American Journal of Clinical Nutrition* 64: 115–119.

———. 2000. Effect of fat adaptation and carbohydrate restoration on metabolism and performance during prolonged cycling. *Journal of Applied Physiology* 89: 2413–2421.

———. 2002. Adaptations to short-term high fat diet persists during exercise despite high carbohydrate availability. *Medicine and Science in Sports and Exercise* 34: 83–91.

Burke, Louise, and Vicki Deakin, eds. 2000. *Clinical Sports Nutrition.* Australia: McGraw-Hill.

Butterfield, G., et al. 1992. Increased energy intake minimizes weight loss in men at high altitude. *Journal of Applied Physiology* 72: 1741–1748.

Campbell, W., et al. 1997. Effects of chromium picolinate and resistance training on body composition in older men. *Medicine and Science in Sports and Exercise* 29 (5) S277.

Carey, A., et al. 2001. Effects of fat adaptation and carbohydrate restoration on prolonged endurance exercise. *Journal of Applied Physiology* 91: 115–122.

Catlin, D. et al. 2000. Trace contamination of over-the-counter androstenedione and positive urine test results for a nandrolone metabolite. *Journal of the American Medical Association* 284: 2618–2621.

Clancy, S., et al. 1994. Effects of chromium picolinate supplementation on body composition, strength and urinary chromium loss in football players. *International Journal of Sport Nutrition* 4: 142–153.

Clarkson, P. 1991. Nutritional ergogenic aids: Chromium, exercise, and muscle mass. *International Journal of Sport Nutrition* 1: 289–293.

———. 1992. Nutritional ergogenic aids: Carnitine. *International Journal of Sport Nutrition* 2: 185–190.

Conley, M., and M. Stone. 1996. Carbohydrate ingestion/supplementation for resistance exercise and training. *Sports Medicine* 21: 7–17.

Coyle, E., et al. 2001. Low-fat diet alters intramuscular substrates and reduces lipolysis and fat oxidation during exercise. *American Journal of Endocrinology and Metabolism* 280: E391–E398.

Davis, J. 1996. Carbohydrates, branched chain amino acids and endurance: The Central Fatigue Hypothesis. *Gatorade Sports Science Exchange* 9 (2).

Decombaz, J., et al. 1993. Effect of L-carnitine on submaximal exercise metabolism after depletion of muscle glycogen. *Medicine and Science in Sports and Exercise* 25: 733–740.

Fallowfield, J., et al. 1995. The influence of ingesting a carbohydrate-electrolyte beverage during 4 hours of recovery on subsequent endurance capacity. *International Journal of Sport Nutrition* 5: 285–299.

Febbraio, M.A., et al. 1996. Carbohydrate feedings before prolonged exercise: Effect of glycemic index on muscle glycogenolysis and exercise performance. *Journal of Applied Physiology* 81: 1115–1120.

Foster-Powell, K., and J. Brand-Miller. 1995. International tables of glycemic index. *American Journal of Clinical Nutrition* 62 (supplement): 871–893.

Graham, T, and L. Spriet. 1996. Caffeine and exercise performance. *Gatorade Sports Science Exchange* 9 (1).

Green, H., et al. 1992. Altitude acclimatization and energy metabolic adaptation in skeletal muscle during exercise. *Journal of Applied Physiology* 73 (6): 2701–2708.

Hellsten-Westing, Y., et al. 1993. Decreased resting levels of adenosine nucleotides in human skeletal muscle after high-intensity training. *Journal of Applied Physiology* 74: 2523–2528.

———1993. The effect of high-intensity training on purine metabolism in man. *Acta Physiologica Scandinavica* 149: 405–412.

Heyward, Vivian H., and Lisa M. Stolarczyk. 1996. *Applied Body Composition Assessment*. Champaign, IL: Human Kinetics.

Ivy, J.L., et al. 1988. Muscle glycogen storage after different amounts of carbohydrate ingestion. *Journal of Applied Physiology* 64 (5): 2018–2023.

———. 1988. Muscle glycogen synthesis after exercise: Effect of time of carbohydrate ingestion. *Journal of Applied Physiology* 64 (4): 1480–1485.

Jendendrup, A., et al. 1997. Carbohydrate-electrolyte feedings improve 1 hour time trial cycling performance. *International Journal of Sports Medicine* 18: 125–129.

Kang, J., et al. 1995. Effect of carbohydrate ingestion subsequent to carbohydrate supercompensation on endurance performance. *International Journal of Sport Nutrition* 5: 329–343.

Kimber, N.E., et al. 2002. Energy balance during an Ironman triathlon in male and female triathletes. *International Journal of Sport Nutrition and Exercise Metabolism* 12: 47–62.

King, D., et al. 1999. Effect of oral androstenedione on serum testosterone and adaptation to resistance training in young men. *Journal of the American Medical Association* 281: 2020–2028.

Kirwan, J.P., et al. 1988. Carbohydrate balance in competitive runners during successive days of intense training. *Journal of Applied Physiology* 65 (6): 2601–2606.

Kovacs, E.M.R., et al. 2002. Effect of high and low fluid intake on post-exercise rehydration. *International Journal of Sport Nutrition and Exercise Metabolism* 12: 14–23.

Kreider, R., et al. 1998. Creatine supplement: Analysis of ergogenic value, medical safety, and concerns. *Journal of Exercise Physiology online* 1 (1): 1–11.

Lambert, E., et al. 2001. High-fat diet versus habitual diet prior to carbohydrate loading: Effects on exercise metabolism and cycling performance. *International Journal of Sport Nutrition and Exercise Metabolism* 11: 209–225.

Lemon, P., et al. 1992. Protein requirements and muscle mass/strength changes during intensive training in novice bodybuilders. *Journal of Applied Physiology* 73: 767–775.

———. 1995. Do athletes need more dietary protein and amino acids? *International Journal of Sport Nutrition* 5: S39–61.

Madsen, K., et al. 1996. Effects of glucose, glucose plus branched-chain amino acids, or placebo on bike performance over 100 km. *Journal of Applied Physiology* 81: 2644–2650.

Mason, W., et al. 1993. Carbohydrate ingestion during exercise: Liquid versus solid feedings. *Medicine and Science in Sport and Exercise* 25: 966–969.

McConnell, G., et al. 1996. Effect of timing of carbohydrate ingestion during exercise performance. *Medicine and Science in Sport and Exercise* 28: 1300–1304.

Millard-Stafford, M., et al. 1992. Carbohydrate-electrolyte replacement improves distance running performance in the heat. *Medicine and Science in Sports and Exercise* 24: 943–940.

Nicholas, C.W., et al. 1997. Carbohydrate intake and recovery of intermittent running capacity. *International Journal of Sport Nutrition* 7: 251–260.

Nissen, S., et al. 1996. Effect of leucine metabolite B-hydroxy-B-methylbutarate on muscle metabolism during resistance training exercise. *Journal of Applied Physiology* 81: 2095–2104.

Parkin, J., et al. 1997. Muscle glycogen storage following prolonged exercise: Effect of timing of ingestion of high glycemic index food. *Medicine and Science in Sport and Exercise* 29: 220–224.

Pascoe, D., and L. Gladden. 1996. Muscle glycogen resynthesis after short term, high intensity exercise, and resistance exercise. *Sports Medicine* 21: 98–118.

Paul, D.R., et al. 2001. Carbohydrate-loading during the follicular phase of the menstrual cycle: Effect on muscle glycogen and exercise performance. *International Journal of Sport Nutrition and Exercise Metabolism* 11: 430–441.

Peters, E., et al. 1993. Vitamin C supplementation reduces the incidence of postrace symptoms of upper-respiratory-tract infection in ultramarathon runners. *American Journal of Clinical Nutrition* 57: 170–174.

Pizza, F., et al. 1995. A carbohydrate loading regimen improves high intensity, short duration exercise performance. *International Journal of Sport Nutrition* 5: 110–116.

Reed, M.J., et al. 1989. Muscle glycogen storage postexercise: Effect of mode of carbohydrate administration. *Journal of Applied Physiology* 66 (2): 720–726.

Rosenbloom, Christine A., ed. 2000. *Sports Nutrition: A Guide for the Professional Working with Active People.* Chicago, IL: The American Dietetic Association.

Roy, B., and M. Tarnopolsky, et al. 1998. Influence of differing macronutrient intakes on muscle glycogen resynthesis after resistance exercise. *Journal of Applied Physiology* 84 (3): 890–896.

Roy, R., et al. 1997. Effect of glucose supplement timing on protein metabolism after resistance training. *Journal of Applied Physiology* 82 (6): 1882–1888.

Ryan, Monique. 1998. *Complete Guide to Sports Nutrition.* Boulder, CO: VeloPress.

Sherman, W.M., et al. 1989. Effects of 4 hour preexercise carbohydrate feedings on cycling performance. *Medicine and Science in Sports and Exercise* 21 (5): 598–604.

———. 1991. Carbohydrate feedings 1 hour before exercise improves cycling performance. *American Journal of Clinical Nutrition* 54: 866–870.

Shirreffs, S., et al. 1996. Post-exercise rehydration in man: Effect of volume consumed and drink sodium content. *Medicine and Science in Sports and Exercise* 28 (10): 1260–1271.

Stanko, R., et al. 1990. Enhanced leg exercise endurance with a high-carbohydrate diet and dihydroxyacetone and pyruvate. *Journal of Applied Physiology* 68: 1651–1656.

———. 1990. Enhancement of arm exercise endurance capacity with dihydroxyacetone and pyruvate. *Journal of Applied Physiology* 68: 119–124.

Tarnolpolsky, Mark, ed. 1999. *Gender Differences in Metabolism*. Boca Raton, FL: CRC Press.

Tarnopolsky, M. A., et al. 2001. Gender differences in carbohydrate loading are related to energy intake. *Journal of Applied Physiology* 91: 225–230.

———. 1997. Postexercise protein-carbohydrate and carbohydrate supplements increase muscle glycogen in men and women. *Journal of Applied Physiology* 83 (6): 1877.

Thompson, D. et al. 2001. Prolonged vitamin C supplementation and recovery from demanding exercise. *International Journal of Sport Nutrition and Exercise Metabolism* 11: 466–481.

Thompson, J., et al. 1996. Effects of diet and diet-plus-exercise programs on resting metabolic rate: A meta-analysis. *International Journal of Sport Nutrition* 6: 41–61.

Tullson, P., and R. Terjung. 1991. Adenine nucleotide synthesis in exercising and endurance-trained skeletal muscle. *American Journal of Applied Physiology* 2651: C342–C347.

Volek, J., and W. Kramer. 1996. Creatine supplementation: Its effect on human and muscular performance and body composition. *National Strength and Conditioning Association, Journal of Strength and Conditioning Research* 10 (3): 200–210.

Walker, L., et al. 1997. Effect of chromium picolinate on body composition and muscular performance in collegiate wrestlers. *Medicine and Science in Sports and Exercise* 29 (5): S278.

Wojcik, J.R., et al. 2001. Comparison of carbohydrate and milk-based beverages on muscle damage and glycogen following exercise. *International Journal of Sport Nutrition and Exercise Metabolism* 11: 406–419.

Yaspelkis, B., et al. 1993. Carbohydrate supplementation spares muscle glycogen during variable-intensity exercise. *Journal of Applied Physiology* 75: 1477–1485.

INDEX

ABOUT THE AUTHOR

Monique Ryan, MS, RD, has been a registered dietitian since 1984 and is the founder of Personal Nutrition Designs, a nutrition consulting company based in the Chicago area. Ryan provides nutrition assessment, education, and counseling to diverse groups of athletes with an emphasis on long-term follow-up and support programming. Ryan has extensive experience in the specialty of sports nutrition and has counseled athletes from the beginner to world class level on how to improve their performance with cutting-edge sports nutrition strategies. Ryan also counsels clients in the areas of weight management, injury rehabilitation, women's health, eating disorder recovery, medical nutrition therapy, and disease prevention and wellness.

Ryan has extensive experience working with endurance athletes. She is the member of the Performance Enhancement Team for USA Triathlon through the 2004 Olympic Games in Athens. She has been the nutritionist for the Saturn Cycling Team since the 1994 season and also consults with the Chicago Fire soccer team. She has also provided nutrition programs for many professional triathletes. Ryan has also been a nutrition consultant for the Volvo-Cannondale Mountain Bike Team, Rollerblade Racing Team, USA Cycling, and the Trek-Volkswagen and Gary Fisher Mountain Bike teams. She has presented to sports nutritionists, coaches, and athletes locally, nationally, and internationally including in Canada, Brazil, and Australia. Her book, *Complete Guide to Sports Nutrition*, is available from VeloPress (1999). Ryan has been quoted frequently in the *Chicago Tribune's* "Training Table" column. For several months in 2000, Ryan was on sabbatical at the Australian Institute of Sport in Canberra, one of the world's top training, physiology, and sports nutrition research centers.

Ryan is the author of more than 150 published articles. Since 1991 she has written sports nutrition articles for *VeloNews*, and also writes for *Inside Triathlon*, and the website for Terry Precision Bicycles. She has also contributed articles to *Triathlete* and *Women's Sports and Fitness*. Ryan has also contributed chapters to *Sports Nutrition: A Guide for the Professional Working with Active People*. She has appeared on CLTV, FOX TV, and the ABC and CBS news. Ryan is a member of the Sports, Cardiovascular, and Wellness Nutritionists (SCAN) practice group and was Reviews Editor of SCAN's quarterly publication, the PULSE, for twelve years. Since 1997, Ryan has been a "Friend of the Team in Training" for the Leukemia and Lymphoma Society. She has participated as a local sponsor and donated workshops for fundraising participants training for marathons, triathlons, and cycling events.

Ryan earned her bachelor of science degree in nutrition and dietetics and completed her clinical training at Northwestern Memorial Hospital Medical Center in Chicago. She also has a master of science in nutrition. Ryan is a member of the American College of Sports Medicine (ACSM) and is an ACSM Health and Fitness Instructor. She has competed in the sports of road cycling and mountain biking.

A description of nutrition programs from Personal Nutrition Designs can be found at www.moniqueryan.com.